Donald Fleming

William H. Welch

and the Rise

of Modern

Medicine

William H. Welch
and the
Rise of
Modern Medicine

Donald Fleming

William H. Welch
and the
Rise of
Modern Medicine

The Johns Hopkins University Press
Baltimore

Copyright © 1954 by Donald Fleming
Copyright © renewed 1982 by Donald Fleming
Afterword copyright © 1987 by The Johns Hopkins University Press
All rights reserved
Printed in the United States of America

Originally published by Little, Brown and Company,
Boston, 1954, as part of the Library of American Biography series,
edited by Oscar Handlin.

Johns Hopkins Paperbacks edition, 1987

The Johns Hopkins University Press
701 West 40th Street
Baltimore, Maryland 21211

Library of Congress Cataloging-in-Publication Data

Fleming, Donald, 1923–
William H. Welch and the rise of modern medicine.

Reprint. Originally published: Boston: Little, Brown, c1954. Originally published in series: The library of American biography.
Includes index.
1. Welch, William Henry, 1850–1934. 2. Physicians—United States—Biography. 3. Medical education—United States—History—20th century. 4. Medicine—United States—History—20th century. I. Handlin, Oscar, 1915– . II. Title. [DNLM: 1. Welch, William Henry, 1850–1934. 2. History of Medicine, 19th Cent.—United States. 3. History of Medicine, 20th Cent.—United States. 4. Physicians—biography. WZ 100 W4417FL 1954a]
R154.W32F5 1987   610'.92'4 [B]   86-46273
ISBN 0-8018-3389-2 (pbk.)

Editor's Preface

PERHAPS even more than other people, Americans have been concerned with the problems of illness and disease. Settlers on a new continent, cut off from traditional remedies and familiar environment, the men of the New World were subject to frequent and unusual maladies; and they spent a good deal of time worrying about the preservation of their health.

Doctors early made an appearance in America, and medicine was a well-established art by the eighteenth century. Whether it did much then to relieve disease or prolong human life is, however, altogether doubtful. Poorly educated and often careless, the early practitioners served their patients largely as a source of psychological comfort. On the other hand, the growth of population and the scarcity of even badly prepared doctors left room for every abuse quacks could contrive. Understandably, most Americans had so little confidence in the art of medicine that they preferred to take their chances with commercial patent-medicine preparations, the variety and abundance of which always astounded foreign travelers.

The decisive change came when American medicine made contact in the late nineteenth century with developments in Europe that were altering the whole nature of the treatment of disease. In the great scientific centers the realization had dawned that medicine depended upon scientific knowledge of the nature and causes of disease. In the clinics and laboratories a new experimental science was developing, largely through the efforts of dedicated men free from the cares of the medical practitioner. These developments had no counterpart, however, in the United States. Neither the universities nor the organized medical societies had the necessary resources or the personnel.

Then, in the last two decades of the nineteenth century came a remarkable transformation. The results of the European investigations, transferred to the United States, were given organized form in medical schools and research institutions. Quickly the whole practice of medicine in the United States changed. The new developments received abundant financial support, and, after the First World War, the world center for the study of medicine shifted to the New World. Since then modern medicine has, in many ways, altered the terms of human existence.

The critical figure in the transformation was William H. Welch, whose life spanned the old and the new medicine. His career illuminates the nature of both the old medicine and the new medicine, and it reveals in a startling and dramatic fashion the sources of modern science and modern education in the United States.

OSCAR HANDLIN

Contents

	Editor's Preface	v
I	Medicine in America	3
II	The New England Background	12
III	New York: the First Phase	24
IV	The Creative Tradition	32
V	New York: the Second Phase	57
VI	The Last Student Days	71
VII	The Johns Hopkins Hospital	77
VIII	A Very Happy Band	96
IX	The Laboratory Regimen in Baltimore	119
X	The Birth of an Influential	131
XI	The Rockefeller Institute	152
XII	Osler and After Osler	161
XIII	The Apotheosis of an Influential	185
	An Afterword, 1987	203
	A Note on the Sources	219
	Acknowledgments	221
	Index	223

William H. Welch
and the
Rise of
Modern Medicine

*To my grandmother and grandfather,
Laura Sipe Beery and Charles Edgar Beery*

I
Medicine in America

WHEN William Henry Welch died in 1934 he left instructions to be buried in his home town of Norfolk, Connecticut. His friend Harvey Cushing spoke of the fitness of his becoming in the end by this symbolic act "just another of the many Doctors Welch of Norfolk" — "all apparently men of very similar type, good judges of people and good public servants, men able to instill confidence and win regard." The great man of his family was subdued to his environment by the elegiac note and reduced to harmony with the quiet and steadiness of the New England village of his birth.

The continuity was deceptive, and the discontinuity profound. The Welch physicians who preceded him were men of charity and consolation, with a genius for conduct rather than thought; he himself became a man of study and of uncomfortable truth-telling, and the spokesman for change and innovation. Compassion, generosity, and kindliness he shared with them, but these were incidental. They helped him to do his work, but did not define or constitute the work. The secret of his career lay in combining a personality that breathed comfort, serenity, and ease, with a deep and overriding intellectual commitment to rebellion against the *status quo* in medicine and medical instruction.

Formal instruction in medicine had begun in America in 1765 with the return of Dr. John Morgan to Philadelphia from his studies in Europe. He then took the lead in founding the first American medical school as part of Benjamin Franklin's College of Philadelphia. In a brilliant inaugural address he laid down the principles on which medical schools ought to be run. The first requirement, he said, was that every graduate should know the whole range of medical science. As late as 1870 a student of the Harvard Medical School could fail four out of nine subjects, secure his degree, and set up practice anywhere in Massachusetts; and one of these doctors on the majority principle killed three successive patients at the beginning of the seventies through ignorance of the lethal dose of morphine.

Morgan said in 1765 that young men should come to the study of medicine able to read Latin, Greek, and French and acquainted with mathematics and the sciences. Before 1900 only one American medical school required a knowledge of French and German and possession of a college degree on entrance; and this school was begun, with misgivings on this score, in 1893.

Morgan said in 1765 that the spirit of the Philadelphia arts faculty, as communicated to the medical school, would help medicine to "put on the form of a regular science." As late as 1912, clinical professors in the Harvard Medical School were chosen on the basis of seniority from among themselves by a group of local physicians, having no status in the university, who met at the Tavern Club in Boston.

Morgan said in 1765 that clinical lectures by physicians of the Pennsylvania Hospital should form an integral part of instruction in the medical school of the College of Philadelphia. The first hospital in Philadelphia and the first important hospital in America built for the purpose of teaching medicine, the University Hospital founded by the younger William Pepper, opened its doors in 1874.

Morgan said in 1765 that medicine could not be learned "without we follow a certain order," from anatomy at the beginning to "praxis" at the end. The first graded sequence of medical studies in America was instituted at Northwestern University in 1859, and the curriculum of the Harvard Medical School was first graded by President Charles William Eliot, over opposition from the faculty, in 1871.

Morgan quoted with approval in 1765 the dictum of the Academy of Surgery of Paris: "We must dive into the bottom of things by repeated and different experiments, and, as it were, force nature to yield herself up to our inquiries." The first laboratory of experimental medicine in America — two rooms in an attic — was begun by the physiologist Henry P. Bowditch, of Harvard, in 1871. One of his colleagues protested against letting students "while away" their time in "the labyrinths of Chemistry and Physiology."

Morgan said in 1765 that his prospective usefulness as a professor in the medical school of Philadelphia required some leisure from an "over hurry" of practice. The first clinical professor in an American medical school who strove to make teaching and research overbalance private consultations was given his great opportunity in 1889. He himself criticized the establishment at the same school in 1913 of the first full-time clinical chairs in America as a scheme for the manufacture of "clinical prigs."

What the founder of the first American medical school

called for in vain in 1765, Welch of Johns Hopkins first brought into being as a balanced whole between 1885 and 1914. Eliot and Bowditch of Harvard, Pepper of Pennsylvania, Gilman and Billings of Johns Hopkins went before; Mall and Osler fell into step; but not they but Welch, by the right choice of precursors, colleagues, and successors and a harmonious response to every great defect of medical instruction in America, transformed American medical schools from the worst to the best in the world in one generation. Yet almost every aspiration realized by Welch was clearly stated by John Morgan more than a century before. The historian of American medicine must ask why the work done by Welch lay open to a man born in 1850, in his prime in 1900, and not yet dead or played out in 1930.

The practice of medicine is a way of making money, a treaty with society, an art and a science. In the eighteenth century, an American who wished to make a business of touching on the lives or property of other people expected to be challenged at inspection barriers of one sort or another where the sanction of the community could be had or withheld in the name of the public welfare. The Age of Jackson, the great destructive but also liberating epoch of the early nineteenth century in America, tore these barriers down and left the will of the individual without check or disguise. In medicine thereafter, proprietary medical schools could operate as profit-making enterprises without any honest scrutiny of candidates for their degree. With this breach of the principle laid down by John Morgan that medical schools ought to be part of universities, and open to the currents of disinterestedness that flow through universities, went the gradual abandonment by the states of any serious effort to license physicians. In the end, only the individual conscience of the private man stood between the will of the proprietors and graduates of most medical schools and the public on which they acted. The superego now floated in mid-air with no institutional props to shore it up.

Though the fundamental vice of the proprietary schools lay in their profit-making character, as a class they were not in fact very profitable, and often the chief inducement to join their faculties was a by-product known in the trade as "the reflex" — consultation fees obtained by a professor on the recommendation of his former students. Since many proprietary schools were hard put to meet their running expenses and keep up mortgage payments on real estate, they lacked the means and the impulse to substitute laboratory instruction for didactic lectures or to introduce research. To do these things, even if the instructors had had any idea how to do them, or why, required endowments on a large scale. These in turn awaited the emergence of the new philanthropy — new in its magnitude, new in its list toward science, and new in its social context.

Few things in the history of the nineteenth and early twentieth centuries cast more light on human nature than the appearance of the "wealth problem" — not the money problem, but the wealth problem, how to spend excess money — among men now set free, beyond any previous conception of freedom, to make as much money as they cared to make, substantially without restraint from church or state. The community no longer sat in judgment on private aims of public consequence. But some of the chief beneficiaries then turned around and rebuilt with their own hands walls between themselves and the attainment of their will, and in their own lifetime handed over their money to be spent for public ends by disinterested men. To have one's own way, direct and unexamined and unsanctified by the consent of others, left after all a void, and opened the way for the philanthropies that made possible the revolution in American medicine led by Welch.

Medical research could not, however, have been subsidized to much purpose till at least a few young men were already looking about for the means to do it, if need be on their own — but somehow. More than anything else, the idea of scientific medicine had to impose itself as a possible career for an *American*. The man who meant to make a career of scientific medicine had to imagine a feasible relationship for himself to the whole shifting range of American society. And the difficulties were not entirely of the imagination. When John Morgan announced in 1765 his intention of practicing physic, but not surgery or pharmacy to save time for study, he was told that this was "to forget that I was born an American." When the great clinician Pierre Louis of Paris urged his American disciple James Jackson, Jr., in 1832, to give four or five years to scientific observation, without practice, the elder Jackson vetoed the plan with regrets. "Because in this country his course would have been so singular, as in a measure to separate him from other men. We are a business doing people. We are new. We have, as it were, but just landed on these uncultivated shores; there is a vast deal to be done; and he who will not be doing, must be set down as a drone." When William H. Welch went from New York to Johns Hopkins in 1884, the note persisted still; he might if he chose throw up the career of a great New York consultant to be "a scientific recluse," but America would get the better of him in the end. "His ideas imbibed in Germany are impractical in our form of government."

In spite of his New York friends, Welch went to Baltimore, for a career like his had come at last to seem just barely conceivable in America. The imagination had learned to live with a possibility from which it had always before cut and run away. The emergence of the graduate school, with the founding of the Johns Hopkins University in 1876, now provided the institutional means by which men might have company in the retreat from money-making into a new monasticism.

Furthermore, scientific medicine began, slowly at first and then more rapidly, to be of some practical use, with what this meant in terms of social sanction for the conduct of research. Some research, in the intervals of other work, there had long been among a few exceptional physicians, of whom Daniel Drake of Cincinnati and W. W. Gerhard of Philadelphia were representative.

In 1796 the boy Daniel Drake had ridden with his father out of the meadowland into the oakland, out of the oakland into the rock and red cedar country, and down to the Blue Licks of Kentucky; imagined the vanished herds of buffalo trampling the grass and the bare earth washing from the rocks, and the buffalo dwarfed by the mammoth sunk in the mud around the Licks; tasted the salt water, watched the vapor rise from the salt furnace, smelled the salt and sulphur smell. Drake never lost, but went on to sharpen and refine, year by year from youth into old age, his feeling for the distinctive local note, and his strong sense of the implication of men in nature. At the end of his life he began to publish his great *Diseases of the In-*

terior Valley of North America (1850–1854), an enormous guidebook to population stocks, water levels, town sites, and cycles of disease along the Mississippi and up its branches — the high-water mark in many ways of medical natural history in America. Maps may now be drawn from Drake's material to show the correlation between malaria and yellow fever and the places where mosquitoes were likely to breed; but the book itself never rose to the level of significant generalization. The natural history temper in medicine was receptive, passive, and recording; not contemptible, because it improved the powers of observation; but not likely to contribute in any very specific way to better practice.

Gerhard of Philadelphia went in the 1830's to study under Louis of Paris, the irresistible magnet who drew men across the Atlantic for a generation to learn the "numerical method" — close observation in the wards and exhaustive autopsies, recorded in tables and subjected to statistical analysis. With this powerful if not yet very subtle instrument, Louis proved the bankruptcy of blood-letting and found the distinctive intestinal lesion of typhoid. To the latter discovery Gerhard added the discrimination of typhoid from typhus in 1836 — the great positive achievement of the school of Louis in America. But better diagnosis could not prevent or cure either disease; and the followers of Louis, the man who took blood-letting from the therapeutic repertory, stood in the public mind for destruction of confidence in old modes of treatment and patient resignation to the absence of anything better. Scientific medicine in this tradition could not look for any widespread public approval.

A kind of geological fault in the history of medicine was

needed to change the situation. The decisive break came in the 1870's and 1880's when Louis Pasteur, not a physician, Robert Koch, not a clinician, and Joseph Lister, the surgeon apostle of Pasteur, first began to loom up in the popular mind as representatives of a new type of scientific medicine — experimental, active, manipulating its data by main force, given to speak not of concomitants and symptoms but causes of disease, and crowned by success in prevention and treatment. What medical natural history and the numerical method could not do, the germ theory of disease did: it gave the scientific man of medicine the prospect of general assent to his chosen way of life. The isolation and singularity of the medical research man in America and elsewhere were bound to grow less from this beginning; and it can scarcely have been altogether a coincidence that this was the moment when William H. Welch fixed upon a new kind of American career and opened the door on the future of American medicine.

I I
The New England Background

It was part of Welch's situation that he contrived to make a clean break with the professional attitudes of his father and grandfather, uncles and great-uncle and still figured as merely the last and greatest of a line of Welch doctors. He was instead the first and last of a new line, and in every fundamental respect one of a kind. The human situation from which he took his departure, and how he became a new sort of man among his people without breaking with them, make up the interest of his ancestry and upbringing.

The American founder of the family, Philip, was shanghaied in 1654 as a boy of eleven in Ireland and sold in Boston harbor as an indentured servant. His great-grandson Hopestill fought in the French and Indian War, marched with Arnold to Quebec in the Revolution, and settled in 1772 as a blacksmith at Norfolk in Litchfield County, Connecticut. Two of his sons became physicians, and the younger, Benjamin, lived to be known as "the beloved physician of Norfolk." Three of Benjamin's sons by his first wife became physicians, and two sons by a second wife, Elizabeth Loveland. The older of these, William Wickham, born in 1818, a graduate of the Yale Medical School who had been apprenticed to one of his half-brothers, married in 1844 Emeline Collin, of Hillsdale, New York. She was then twenty-two, a woman of brains and schooling and some wit but no beauty, who wore her hair braided on top, parted in the middle in front, and hanging down in ropes before her ears — one of the harsh, ungainly faces of the first generation of women to sit for the camera.

Shortly after her marriage she went into some sort of physical decline, accompanied by self-reproaches for being ill and a steady increase in piety, and culminating in a deathbed request that her husband build an altar in the home. He was not then or ever a man to build altars. Before her death in October 1850, Emeline Welch bore two children, Emeline, always known as Emma, in 1847, and William Henry on April 8, 1850. Of her influence, it can only be said that she gave her husband a chance to perfect under fire an unshakable passivity in religious matters and then left him to bring up a pair of orphans who had no recollection of ever having a mother.

The grandmother, Elizabeth Loveland Welch, had lived with her son and daughter-in-law throughout their marriage and now took charge of the baby William Henry. His sister Emma was sent to live with some of her mother's people in a nearby town and never again lived regularly in her father's house. The family in Norfolk therefore consisted of the old grandmother, the widowed husband, and the boy. Elizabeth Welch, a handsome woman with a full face and the lawn cap of a woman over forty, was a public figure, the lady superintendent of the Congregational Sunday School and the amateur social worker of the town, who visited the sick and in general went, bearing advice but also something hot in a basket, to help out in times of trouble. When she finally had to give up her work with the Sunday school, she wrote: "I find to part with its special cares is too nearly akin to parting with those of my own beloved Family!" She had in fact a weak sense for the dividing line between family and not family, and by spreading her maternal impulses with an even hand over the whole community ended as a kind of universal grandmother — "Grandma Welch" of Norfolk.

Her son William Wickham Welch, a clear-eyed man with a low-hanging beard, also belonged to the public and oriented his life outward toward the community rather than toward his family. He was always in arrears by half a day or so with his mother and son and the rest of the town, rising toward noon, slow to dispose of his outdoor patients, and late, very late, in setting out on his rounds. His patients came to expect that even on routine calls of no urgency he might arrive in the middle of the night. The fact that a man who lived out of step with the basic rhythms of the community was trusted implicitly as a physician and sent repeatedly to the Connecticut legislature and once, as a Republican, to the United States House of Representatives throws some light on the impact of his personality. With the hours that he kept and his incapacity to wrest any free time for himself from the demands of his practice, the elder Welch even more than other physicians was something of a stranger in the life of his son. "His love of humanity made all as dear to him as were his own household."

There is no reason to think that the boy felt cheated by the climate of diffuse benevolence in which his father and grandmother lived. But he grew up without the right of secure or privileged possession in any other human personality near at hand. He began to correspond with his sister at an early age, and they built up between them an image of the mother whom neither of them could remember. Yet this correspondence of itself was a kind of danger signal of the emotional poverty of his immediate contacts. Though he lived next door to a houseful of cousins and went in and out of their house at will, some final element of assurance was lacking even in this relationship; for he moved a large pile of stones so that his cousins would call him "brother," and they did — for a while. But if a tragedy was going forward, of the boy's not learning to love or be loved and be at rest in the knowledge, it was a tragedy without crises, and he lived on the surface a pleasant enough existence, in which love was not so much withheld as spread thin and undiscriminated. Some mutilation of the personality his mature life disclosed. Meanwhile the quiet village life flowed on, an idyll of its kind, with games on the village green, picnics in "the old spring lot," and in the foreground church and school.

Welch attended a dame school of the old type, kept by two sisters, the Misses Nettleton, who taught the usual things plus sewing for both sexes. The students recited verses from the Bible every day, and cannot have found the tone of their daily instruction very different from that of the Sunday-school lesson supervised by Grandma Welch. But life on Sunday had a consistency that the Misses Nettleton were powerless to impose on weekdays; Sunday school and church might let out, but the church tone must not let up, and Welch recalled that the only licensed recreation was an afternoon walk to the graveyard.

Day in and day out he himself had the special responsibility of being the grandson of a village priestess of the

Puritan sort. If he brought his friends home to play they had to break off on the word that Elizabeth Welch had gone to her bedroom to pray — and she was much given to praying. But the pervasive religious note of life in Norfolk was not oppressive or deadening to the spirit of the children. One of Welch's schoolmates at a later period was described in one breath as a gay fellow, "a Christian and member of the church."

To accept the religious orientation of village life in New England, and not to kick against the traces, was one thing. To make the affirmative response to religion still required of young people in Welch's boyhood was another. By his membership in almost the last generation of children expected to have the conversion experience of New England tradition, he stood at one of the great dividing points in the history of adolescence in America. The divide lay just ahead, not behind, and even the last attenuation of Puritanism imposed a strain. The situation was given a final twist for Welch by the circumstance that though his grandmother and sister were eager that he experience grace, his father never joined the church and suggested to his son, not by precept but by example, the possibility of retreating into inaction and unconcern.

This was not easy for a boy in Welch's position; and the pressure upon him to make manifest his election to grace increased with his transfer at the age of thirteen to a boarding school run by a clergyman uncle. The experience of grace was not, strictly speaking, a thing to be had by trying; but in practice — and more or less in theory — this rather delicate theological issue had been resolved long before in favor of straining after grace as hard as possible. Welch's sister Emma, who had gone on to Mount Holyoke, wrote repeatedly of her hopes for him; and those of his classmates who had not already passed triumphantly through the crisis were in the same state of expectancy, praying for one another, and looking for a sign. They were also riding ponies, hunting rabbits, and indulging in various kinds of horseplay, and the surviving accounts give no impression of gloom or solemnity. Indeed, in the absence of organized athletics, winning through to grace had some of the interest of a sporting event. Who would make the team?

Welch was rather slow to take fire, but he was able to announce before his classmates in March 1864 that he had had the conversion experience. "There is indeed a great revival going on here," he wrote to Emma. "I think about one hundred have expressed their determination of serving the Lord. Among them myself the reason I did not tell you was I was afraid I could not hold out but Emma I do mean to try and I hope I shall have an interest in your prayers that I may not falter and turn back." Emma replied that he ought to tell their father: "I am sure he will be very much rejoiced." Welch refused to be drawn out into conjectures on this score and replied, "I have not yet written father of my hope." The boy did not finally join the church till May 1865.

The initiation rites by which a New England boy might short the circuit to maturity were now accomplished; and Welch, at fifteen, had a station among men and under God. This sliding scale of maturity of the Puritan tradition made it possible for their parents and teachers to provoke a crisis of belief among children and see the fever through to a definitive conclusion, but bore with it its own risks. If the climax of religion came in youth, the discoveries still to be made would lie elsewhere, and maturity might seem to consist in leaving religion behind. In the year 1865 the great issue could not be resolved forever by the age of fifteen.

The grandmother who had followed the boy's spiritual progress so intently was now winding up her affairs, retiring from the Sunday school, and retreating, a semi-invalid, to her bedroom. It can scarcely have been an accident that William Wickham Welch chose this moment to marry again and so administer a severe shock to his son and daughter — "so soon" Emma called it; their mother had then been dead sixteen years. At forty-six, the bride, Emily Sedgwick, was a year younger than her husband. "I don't see," her stepson-to-be wrote, "anything attractive about her without it is her eyes and curls which are certainly striking." But the stranger went quietly on her way, poking into cupboards, planning to knock doors through walls, and confronting her stepchildren with the intolerable problem of what to call her — but not Mother. The blow was softened for Welch by his being busy and happy at school and looking forward to entering Yale. In the end the only fault that he and Emma could find with Emily Welch was a certain sharpness toward her rather disorganized and unsystematic husband. She proved a faithful ally of William Henry Welch when he came to choose a career.

At the age of sixteen Welch entered Yale College — the old somnolent Yale which shut its ears as much as possible against the jarring local note of the Sheffield Scientific School. But education lay in the interstices of the curriculum, and Welch read as a freshman one of the last books he ought to have read by the lights of New Haven orthodoxy, the Bible of geographical determinism in history, Buckle's *History of Civilization*. Sixty years later

Welch was eager that young people should come by their Buckle early: ". . . it had great influence on me." But apparently his immediate response was to sense danger and try to beat it down. "There never was an age," he wrote in an undergraduate essay entered for a prize, "so profoundly hostile to the supernatural, the essence of all religions. The struggle is no longer about Christian dogmas but about the very foundation of Christianity, faith in the unseen and the eternal." Did it not, he asked, "make life hopeless and not worth living" to think of the world as "a vast machine unguided by a God of justice?"

Welch returned in a somewhat lower key to the same theme in a graduating address. The living source of the problem was science, which furthered the "idea of the government of the world by laws, immutable, inexorable." Welch undertook to refute the position that there was nothing beyond nature's laws by vindicating the effectiveness of free will. His argument was well received in the college founded by emigration from Harvard to keep the milk of the word of Calvin from being diluted. But to help to find the laws, and break the back of the abnormal and capricious, had its own fascination and brought its own repose, and Welch had not yet had done with these issues. Buckle might or might not prevail in the end over Grandma Welch. The decision was still in suspense, and being in suspense had already gone against the conversion mechanism of the Congregational Church. Maturity must wait upon the calendar.

Nothing in Welch's life at Yale pointed toward a career either in science or in theology; his real enthusiasm was for the classics. He kept up this interest for some time to come and thought of keeping it up for life, but the critical part of his experience at Yale seems to have been membership in Skull and Bones, the society with no windows, no acknowledged name before men, and no place on the lips of its members in the outside world. Welch always took the view of this distinction to be expected of a Yale man. Many years later when his nephew was looking about for a college, Welch wrote that any number of places would do for the man who could not make Bones, but only one for the man who could. The Yale system of secret societies, with their tradition of keeping a hold on alumni, including members of the faculty, was one of the most powerful engines ever contrived for raising undergraduates above the level of adolescence and depressing graduates below the level of maturity. In this middling atmosphere of warm complicity between coming men and men who had come, some of the business of Yale College was transacted in Welch's time in New Haven. His first conscious impulse toward an academic career sprang from sitting in judgment as a Bones man on instructors and courses at Yale. If his later opinions were any index, Welch thought that much of the instruction in his time was contemptible. The dam burst and swept the old Yale away after he graduated; but of at least one man, E. L. Godkin of *The Nation* was apparently mistaken in charging that the chief drag on the improvement of the college was the influence of Bones.

In 1870 Welch graduated as third man in his class and delivered his oration on science and religion. He knew what he wanted to do next, to stay at Yale as tutor in Greek, "a subject which I think gave me more satisfaction than any other which I studied in college." The only opening in the classics went, however, to one of his friends, and Welch spent a dispirited summer at home in Norfolk hoping for something to turn up. At the very last minute in the fall, he got, through his Yale connections, a chance to teach Cicero and German in an academy in Norwich, New York. This job petered out in the spring of 1871, and Welch once more confronted the problem of a career.

At this low point in his prospects and in his confidence in himself, he turned at last to medicine — not a first choice but the last resort of a man thwarted in his ambition and beaten down by circumstances into conforming with the family tradition. He had held back because he had no desire at all to continue his father's work; and he only began to be happy and successful in medicine as the possibility opened out before him of a new kind of career with no precedent among the Doctors Welch and not much precedent in history.

William Henry Welch grew up unable to bear the sight of blood and the sight and sound of pain, and disturbed by sick people flowing through the house in the daytime and sending messengers to beat on the door at night. He said later that his father had been of no use in giving him any real insight into medicine. But no tutelage would have enabled him to bear patiently with the tide of people in pain that caught a country practitioner up and bore him along through life and never let him go till he died. This side of medicine Welch never found congenial. His father could give him no initiation into the other side, of health and disease as a field of research.

William Wickham Welch was altogether cut off from the great innovating current in American medicine in his time, the therapeutic nihilism and "numerical method" of the French clinician Louis. Osler's "Alabama Student"

John Bassett, who died in 1851, spoke for the school of Louis in America when he said that the physician was never reduced to "dealing a blow in the dark" — "where there are no intelligible indications, it is clear that there should be no action." He added that, in spite of this, "dying men will have pills and parsons." The elder Welch made such pills and lives in memory mixing potions in a bowl, like the more intuitive kind of cook, and tasting for the proportions. He did not feel even at second hand the influence of Louis. Neither did he belong to the traditions of medical natural history, like Daniel Drake. In a third region where American men of medicine were striking out in new directions and trenching at least on science — in surgery — Welch disliked to operate and showed no great skill. His place in the community was not that of a scientist but of a repository of public confidence — the man not of intellect but of character.

Through the summer and fall of 1871 William Henry Welch worked as an apprentice in his father's office. He later chose to talk as if this experience had never been, and his correspondence with Emma and his classmates fell off and touched only in passing on his apprenticeship. He cannot have been happy and may have been miserable. The way out came with his father's blessing: as he had had no science to speak of in college, he must go back to Yale, not the college but the Sheffield Scientific School, and take a course in chemistry. The Sheffield School was not intended for the training of physicians as such, and it was symbolic for Welch's career in medicine that his first formal instruction with a view to this career came not in a school of medicine but of science; and a school visibly passing over in his time from the ideal of practical training for agriculture, industry, and mining to that of disinterested research in pure science — from the ideal of the technical consultant Benjamin Silliman, Sr., to the ideal of the genius of thermodynamics Willard Gibbs. The younger Welch maintained the family tradition only by breaking with it. He could not be subdued in life, and ought not to be subdued in history, to the environment from which he came.

I I I
New York: the First Phase

IN FEBRUARY 1872 Welch was back where he had wished to be ever since he left college, in New Haven — "not much changed" but then again "quite different." "Things look a little more serious and it hardly seems as if I could enjoy the same frolics I delighted in when in college." He took a laboratory course in analytical chemistry in the Sheffield School and heard George F. Barker, one of the better physical scientists of his time in America, lecture at the medical school on F. A. Kekulé's conception of the carbon atom.

Welch had now made his entry into science. He had also purchased his psychological discharge from Yale; because he had found that it would not hold still for him to cling to and because he was now in earnest about medicine, and even Yale men did not go to the Yale Medical School if they could help it. After he had left Yale, never to return except for visits, he received in 1873 the offer for which he would once have given anything, to be a tutor in Greek. He turned it down without hesitation.

In the fall of 1872 Welch entered the College of Physicians and Surgeons in New York. Legally, but hardly more than legally, a part of Columbia College, Physicians and

NEW YORK: THE FIRST PHASE 25

Surgeons was the oldest and best and most arrogant of the three quarrelsome medical schools in New York City. The others were that of New York University — actually a proprietary school which bought diplomas from the university — and the Bellevue Hospital school. If the "University" and Bellevue schools were inferior to their great rival, this was not because Physicians and Surgeons had raised a standard to which the wise and foresighted could repair. It was a good school of a bad kind, a business enterprise with no admission requirements, an ungraded course, a single examination at the end of a man's studies, and a healthy respect for Gresham's law of proprietary medical schools — not to raise one's standards very far above the level of one's worst rival because there would be no standard to maintain if the students took their fees elsewhere. All three schools had some exceptional men on their faculties in Welch's time as a student: the elder Austin Flint at Bellevue, John W. Draper, one of the ablest and most versatile men of science of this and the preceding generation in America, at New York University, and Edward C. Seguin at Physicians and Surgeons. Welch liked to say that the system produced better results and attracted better men to study and teach than anyone had a right to expect; and it certainly produced in him its own nemesis.

When he entered the College of Physicians and Surgeons, of the three parts into which medical instruction was later divided — formal lectures, clinics for the observation of patients, and laboratories — the third scarcely existed, and a man could skimp on clinics. Attendance at the lectures and the religious taking or at any rate the purchasing of lecture notes and committing them to memory was the heart of the program. Welch, however, got his chief stimulus from Edward C. Seguin's clinic for nervous diseases; and from the one enduring laboratory tradition of the medical schools of the Western world from the thirteenth century forward, human dissection. Seguin, a pioneer in introducing the clinical thermometer into American practice, the French-born son of French parents, came to the United States as a boy and only returned to France for graduate study under the physiologist Charles E. Brown-Séquard and the neurologist Jean Charcot. The golden age of French science was then breaking off in a jagged way; but one of the traditions with the most projective force into the future was the neurology of Charcot, Seguin's master — Charcot, from whom Sigmund Freud later heard the shattering aside, "But, in this kind of case, it is always something genital — always, always, always!"

Of this insight Welch almost certainly heard nothing from Seguin. But Seguin modeled his clinics after Charcot's. "No clinics I have ever attended," Welch later wrote, "worked so systematically." "We were in the midst of Charcot's best work, and it interested me enormously." Welch was first induced to follow these clinics by Seguin's offer of a microscope — the thing he then wanted "more than anything else" — for the best notes taken by a student. Welch won the prize, but he had no idea how to use it and waited a long time to find out. Meanwhile he kept it in his room, a constant reminder of what he still had to do to come merely abreast of his generation in Europe, of the necessity for running to stand still.

Welch, who had a low opinion of the average medical student, thought that his own performance was overpraised; but his record brought him an appointment in the fall of 1873 as prosector to the professors of anatomy.

Welch as a boy disliked blood and pain; and as a man he had to get over an initial revulsion from the work of the dissecting room. But in a short time he was busy "night and day" and fascinated by his duties as prosector. In his old age he said that he never felt so proud in his life as when he marched in with the professor and saw his own dissections displayed before the class. This work was the nearest thing to a laboratory course that the college afforded, and for its sake Welch cut many lectures.

On the urging of one of the anatomy professors with whom he thus came in close contact, Welch competed for the chief honor within the gift of the medical faculty, the "thesis prize." His summary of the literature on goiter involved much research in libraries and easily won. A professor in the Bellevue school offered to help pay the costs of publication, one of the pleasant little gestures of good will that almost never happened among the embattled medical faculties of New York City. But Welch had already thrown bridges across from Physicians and Surgeons to Bellevue and, a real feat of cultural engineering, from both to New York University by taking courses at the despised and despising rival schools. In spite of the extra work, Welch as a student found a little time for church, some time for art galleries and fashionable shops, much time for music — spectator's music, operas and concerts — but scarcely any time for young women. Except for his stepmother, whom he had come to like and respect, the only woman who meant anything to him was his sister Emma, now a married woman of several years standing, whose husband Stuart Walcott was on intimate terms with Welch.

Before his graduation in February 1875, Welch had already received an appointment as intern at Bellevue Hospital and had begun to work but not to live there. After graduation he became a resident and met the usual crises with at least usual success. At Bellevue he came within the orbit of a remarkable man, the pathologist Francis Delafield, still young but already one of the great "dead house" men of his time in America — a commanding figure in the hospital morgues. From the school of Louis, Delafield had learned to check the clinical diagnosis against the autopsy — always — and to enter in his notebook the raw materials for the statistical analysis of disease also commended by Louis. From the newer tradition of Rudolf Virchow, Delafield had learned in addition to regard the cells as the building blocks of anatomy and the ultimate sites of malformation and malfunction. Life had become for Delafield at bottom a tireless salting away of new instances in his locally famous "book"; and he seemed very remote from his colleagues and students. Welch would watch him in his black skullcap and ticking apron, his austerity a little relieved by a meerschaum pipe, cutting and staining sections and looking at them under the microscope. In spite of his eagerness to bring his own inert possession to life, Welch looked on wistfully and never ventured to ask Delafield for instruction in how to use a microscope.

Delafield singled out Welch for the great distinction of making entries of his own cases directly in the "book" and of filling in during the summer vacation of 1875 as curator of pathological specimens at Bellevue. This was the tribute of an intellect to an intellect; but another friend of Welch at Bellevue, the German refugee of 1848 Abraham Jacobi, the real founder of pediatrics in the United States, fixed on other qualities. Welch, he said, not only "leaked" knowledge to his colleagues, without being obtrusive about it, but showed himself modest and gentle in treating the sick. "I then felt certain that he would be a great physician or practitioner, whose make-up always requires, though it does not always furnish, head and heart."

Welch had now graduated from one of the best colleges and one of the best medical schools and worked with one of the best pathologists, perhaps the best of all, in the country. He had gone in fact almost as far as America would take him. He had at home no prospect of growth except to be his own master and perfect himself slowly in active practice over the years, with teaching as a possible adjunct. But ever since his undergraduate days at Yale he had been inclined to think of teaching as a sufficient career in itself, and he now saw looming immediately ahead the one opportunity of his generation in America to teach medicine for the sake of teaching medicine. There was no time to ripen by self-education into a plausible candidate.

Johns Hopkins, a Quaker merchant of Baltimore and a bachelor, died in 1873. He left behind him the largest philanthropic bequest of American history up to that time, about $7,000,000, for the establishment of a university and a hospital, with a medical school to serve as a link between them. Ezra Cornell had already launched the second founding age of universities in America, touched with gold like nothing in the history of education anywhere ever before. But Cornell University, first opened in 1868, had been a disappointment to some people. The opportunity to revolutionize higher education still lay open to the Johns Hopkins University and its first president Daniel Coit Gilman.

Gilman was a product of the only vigorous native tradition of graduate schooling, a tradition mixed up with the founding and growth of the Sheffield School at Yale. In his new position he gave promise of being the revolutionary for whom some Americans, Welch among them, were looking. By 1875 Welch had learned that the projected medical school intended to further basic research, and he had begun to dream of filling the chair of pathological anatomy. He had never met Gilman in New Haven, but his best friend Frederic Dennis undertook to act as intermediary. Dennis, the son of a wealthy father, had gone to boarding school with Welch in Connecticut, had followed him to Yale and the College of Physicians and Surgeons, and had determined to be king-maker for his friend. In the summer of 1875 he went to Europe on the same boat with Gilman and seized the opportunity to talk about Welch, who said, however, that it was "folly for me to aspire to attaining such a position when there are so many distinguished men in the country who have already acquired great reputations as pathologists."

In spite of these protestations Welch went to the trouble of calling on Gilman in Baltimore late in 1875 — without, however, seeing him — and took an indulgent view of Dennis's rather high-pressure tactics for bringing "the Yale influence" to bear. But Welch knew that the warrant that Gilman sought was not New Haven, or New York or Philadelphia, but Berlin or Leipzig. Dennis was going abroad to study; the elder Dennis offered to get Welch passage at half-fare and ended by making up the other half; Emma and Stuart Walcott were enthusiastic and offered a loan of $500; and the united voice of Welch's teachers said to go. William Wickham Welch, who would have to foot most of the bill for living abroad, had been looking forward to the return of his only son to Norfolk as a partner. But he yielded without real resistance. His wife, the once-dreaded stepmother, was favorable from the beginning.

On April 19, 1876, William Henry Welch embarked on the great adventure of his life. He would now have the chance to meet some of the great men in medicine, to get the feel of the current situation in science, and to try his hand at genuine research. In the process he would find himself at the center of the distinctive intellectual experiment of his time, the effort being made by the Germans to produce a steady flow of creative investigators in science.

IV
The Creative Tradition

THE MOST AUDACIOUS enterprise of the nineteenth century may well have been the effort to organize a creative tradition in science; to make systematic the emergence of intellects hostile to system, routine, and tradition. The only true analogue in modern times was the artist's studio of the High Renaissance, half workshop for journeymen apprentices and half forcing-ground for genius.

Before the nineteenth century the experiments, largely unconscious, in the production of creative intellects in science would stop and start and stop again, spring up and die away, without flowing together into a continuous tradition. The men who founded and worked in the pioneer laboratories of the nineteenth century made a new departure. There the unteachable was taught and the succession of genius prolonged.

The chief thing the master had to give to his best students — and got from them in return — was a nagging malaise and the likelihood of being thrown off balance and spun around and made unhappy with previous efforts and assumptions. This accessibility to shock, the need for an irreducible minimum of friction, strain, and unsubmissiveness in the relationship between master and student, marked the first encounter, in 1827, between the future embryologist Karl Ernst von Baer and his chosen teacher Ignaz Döllinger — as good an emblem as any of the beginnings of the effort to teach creativity in science. Of this first exchange, with Döllinger's brushing aside the kind of thing that von Baer had come for and off-handedly taking for granted that he could and would do things that he did not even know how to begin to do, the younger man said, "I was thunderstruck," and the charm was wound up. Von Baer bought a leech from a pharmacist and began to cut it up slowly and clumsily, until Döllinger was ready with his next careless blow and took down from the shelves a monograph which showed how to do the thing right. The whole experience was symbolic of the strategy of letting the student work himself into corners and holding back, what had to be held back until it came a little late, the ready-made solution and the easy hint. Into this rich human and historical situation Welch was now beginning to feel his way. That was the meaning of his stay in Europe.

Welch went first to Strassburg, now a German university from which every trace of French influence had been removed. For him the special attraction there was the presence of the pathological anatomist F. D. von Recklinghausen. But von Recklinghausen took only advanced students who were skilled in the use of the microscope; and this excluded Welch. He therefore studied normal histology under Wilhelm Waldeyer, in preparation for future work with von Recklinghausen. At the same time, in the spring and early summer of 1876, Welch also studied under E. F. Hoppe-Seyler, the founder of physiological chemistry as a separate discipline.

In August he moved on to Leipzig, with the intention

of working with the authority on nervous diseases, Johann Heubner — apparently a last echo of the deep impression made by Seguin. Heubner, however, was marking time till he could effect a transfer to another field. To fill up the vacuum Welch enrolled under the physiologist Carl Ludwig, and under Ludwig's stimulus made a discovery of some importance in anatomy. In Leipzig, Welch also improved his microscopic technique under the pathologist Ernst Wagner, and attended the lectures of Rudolf Leuckart on comparative anatomy.

In April 1877 Welch went to Breslau, where he worked in the laboratory of the pathologist Julius Cohnheim and carried through by far the most important investigation of his career to date. Here he came in contact also with Cohnheim's assistant Carl Weigert. Perhaps as a sop to his father — and his own conscience — Welch attended three clinics in Breslau. But in Vienna, the home of the machine-produced clinician, he spent the month of October 1877 not in attending clinics but learning embryology in the laboratory of F. von Schenck. In December, Welch was back in Strassburg to pursue a piece of investigation under von Recklinghausen. He sailed for America in February 1878.

This catalogue of names, dates, and fields of study can only be brought to life in terms of the initiation into creativity for which they stood in Welch's mind — the concrete exemplification of an experiment in which he and his teachers and fellow students were engaged in common.

Welch and others stood to gain three things from the graduate training given in Germany: a first entry into a new political structure of great interest and delicacy; an *interested* initiation into the present state of scientific opinion, so that scientific controversies were invested with personal overtones of the men who had something at stake in the outcome; and finally an introduction to possible themes, methods, and purposes of research.

Science as a domain of politics, an arena for the exercise of power, found its place within the structure of politics at large. Of the three great scientific peoples of the nineteenth century, the English alone combined a maximum of freedom in the state, freedom in society at large, and freedom in the conduct of science — with the exception of certain restraints imposed by Parliament on animal vivisection. But science in England tended, more than elsewhere, to be the concern of an anarchic community of brilliant amateurs and private men, lacking in articulation and cohesion.

With the French and the Germans the issue was more complicated. The French thought of themselves, and were thought of, as a freedom-loving people; and at least in Paris they gave to themselves and others an unparalleled sense of elbowroom in the conduct of life. But they maintained under all regimes the policy of rigid control of the provincial administration from Paris. As part of the process by which Paris sucked France dry, the provincial universities were deprived of all local initiative and deliberately subordinated to the Sorbonne and the Collège de France. In science, as elsewhere, the faculties of the provincial universities were divided between apathetic men of the second rank who could not hope for Paris or for dignity and prestige anywhere else and driving men of the first rank who were fighting their way toward Paris. Of the brilliant chemist Charles Gerhardt, Wilhelm Ostwald said that his career might be summed up in the single phrase, The Battle for Paris; and, after all, the call never came. Gerhardt had a vindictive enemy at the Sorbonne, and a man who wished to re-emerge from exile in the provinces could not afford to antagonize the men in possession.

The authoritarian strain in the public institutions of the French had communicated itself to the polity of French science; and to this among other considerations one must look for an explanation of the increasing superiority of German science to French as the nineteenth century wore on. Apart from the special case of Charles Darwin, the half-dozen greatest names in nineteenth-century biology were equally divided between the two peoples: Georges Cuvier, Claude Bernard, Louis Pasteur; Johannes Müller, Rudolf Virchow, and Robert Koch. But among men on the next level, the Germans predominated by far. They had, and the French had not, the art of producing creative investigators in depth. If only for the chance of learning this art Welch had done well to go to Germany.

It was symbolic of the difference between France and Germany that Welch on his first visit to Germany did not study in Berlin at all, and found great men like von Recklinghausen, Ludwig, and Cohnheim content to spend the rest of their lives in Strassburg, Leipzig, and Breslau. He could easily have found other men of comparable distinction in still other universities. The fact that Berlin never became in the nineteenth century the Paris of Germany gave to many scientists in many places psychological repose and some measure of relief from academic climbing. Even the greatest scholars in Germany could not dominate and tyrannize over the whole body of their fellow investigators without restraint; because, in contrast to France, in any given field of research there was not a single unified polity controlled from the center but a loose federation of polities.

The long delay in securing the political unification of Germany was regarded by the bulk of enlightened opinion throughout the Western world as a grave misfortune. Instead it was an incalculable advantage and helped to make possible the distinctive role of the Germans in history: to have built in the realm of scholarship and science a new structure of power of which the law was freedom and noncoercion. Science became the enclave of freedom in German society, and the ultimate repository of the liberal impulses which had seemed to reach their climax in 1848 and die away. The sense that with advanced students only the lightest kind of supervision could be tolerated went very deep in the greater German scientists and characterized most if not all of the men who succeeded in arousing creativity in others. To learn the uses of freedom in the teaching of science — to share in the conquest of a new area for the exercise of freedom — Englishmen, Frenchmen, and Americans alike had to go to Germany. The immersion of William Henry Welch in this atmosphere therefore became a significant event in the history of liberty in America.

Of the three men with whom he chiefly studied during his first stay in Germany — von Recklinghausen of Strassburg, Ludwig of Leipzig, and Cohnheim of Breslau — Welch found that von Recklinghausen practiced an almost total want of supervision. "He bestows very little personal attention upon those working with him." But sometimes he would talk with Welch about current problems in pathology, and convey some of the barely articulate wisdom that craftsmen of all kinds transmit by word of mouth or not at all. In his strategy of standing largely aloof from the work being done in his laboratory, von Recklinghausen had some company among the more successful teacher-investigators of the nineteenth century. Of the great cytologist Wilhelm His, one of his American pupils later wrote: "All of the details were left to the pupil and it annoyed him to be consulted regarding them. He desired that the pupil should have full freedom to work out his own solution and aided him mainly through severe criticism." Abuses of power can always be avoided by abdication of power; and a near approach to abdication was the temperamentally congenial solution for men like His and von Recklinghausen.

The real test of the commitment to freedom for one's students came with men who held power and wielded it; and above all men holding and wielding power who had the outgoing personality that wished to lose its identity in being helpful to others. The type of this personality among the biologists of the nineteenth century was Welch's teacher at Leipzig, Carl Ludwig, the founder of the most flourishing school of physiologists of his time and the successor to John Hunter of London at the end of the eighteenth century and Louis of Paris in the middle of the nineteenth as the favorite teacher abroad of the abler American students of medicine.

Ludwig presided over the best-known and most elaborate physiological institute in Europe. Dedicated in 1869, it was a miniature world of his own, the Museum of Alexandria and the Grand Hotel rolled into one, with stables, kennels, and rabbit hutches, frog ponds and fish ponds, workshops, laboratories, and lecture rooms, and living quarters for himself and others. He also had subjects to govern: pampered mechanics, carpenters, and technicians, *Dienern* to fetch and carry and clean up and air out, undergraduates returning semester after semester to get the sense of his difficult lectures, advanced students like Welch pursuing their researches, and assistant professors of chemistry and microscopic anatomy waiting their turn to move upward on the academic ladder. Unlike His and von Recklinghausen, Ludwig kept close watch over everything in the institute. "Ludwig is a charming man," Welch wrote, "and the air of the whole place is the most cheerfully scientific of any laboratory I have ever been in."

Welch's contemporaries spoke of the contagious joy with which Ludwig, *Menschenfreund,* with beaked nose and long hair, would make his rounds every morning with the question, "Well, what's new today?" The night before he would have taken "home" to his living quarters the records of the various current investigations and studied them in preparation for his tour of the next day; he was then ready to discuss for a few minutes in passing what the investigator proposed to do next, or if necessary to take him off for a long private conference in which methods, assumptions, and conclusions would be threshed out. Of the tags of wisdom and bits of philosophy that it was the business of Ludwig to throw out and wise students to treasure up, one has been preserved: "It is not good to have too many ideas."

Ludwig was proof by nature against the temptation to abuse his power by domineering over his associates and repressing dissent. But he was guilty of the more insidious fault, to which his good qualities laid him open, of depriving students of freedom for their own benefit. There are many stories of his and his technician's carrying through to completion investigations planned by himself and given over to the student to publish in the student's name. His admirers said that he gave proof in this way of selflessness, but within the polity of science it was the selflessness that paralyzes and devours — from generous motives. Yet nothing of this kind happened with Welch and other men of his ability; and they took away with them the prevailing sense of freedom which Ludwig had spread about him in the most difficult of circumstances — moving constantly among his students and wishing out of good nature to do their work for them.

Julius Cohnheim of Breslau, a handsome blond still in his thirties, was a middle term between the two extremes of von Recklinghausen and Ludwig. He came to the laboratory "very often, though not daily," proposed subjects for investigation, and for the benefit of Welch's best friend in Breslau, the Dane Carl Salomonsen, set up general inoculation tuberculosis in guinea pigs. But by the time of Welch's arrival Cohnheim had ceased to be greatly interested in pathological anatomy, and had substantially handed the field over to his brilliant assistant Carl Weigert.

With this retreat went a mild skepticism about the new methods of staining sections and the importance attached to staining in general. Welch had brought with him from New York Francis Delafield's haematoxylin stain, and Cohnheim insisted that use be made of this in the ordinary instruction which fell to Weigert. But there was a mocking undertone to his question, often repeated, "What are you painting today, Herr Welch?" "But you are really a master dyer!" he would say ironically in turn to all of the young men who shared in the new enthusiasm.

By Welch's day much of the work of the laboratory had

slipped away from Cohnheim, partly by choice and partly by the onrush of new techniques which he could not and would not exclude from his institute but would never find wholly congenial. Yet Cohnheim remained productive and a genius, and intellectually if not emotionally receptive to new ideas; and Welch saw in its least tragic form the process of the leaving behind of the master by his own students. In this sense freedom for the oncoming generation in science need not be with von Recklinghausen an abdication of power or with Ludwig a gift deliberately bestowed, but merely the supersession of the old by the young and the young by the younger. But freedom in the laboratory was not simply a trick played upon Cohnheim by Nature. Where he undertook to participate in the work of his students, mainly by suggesting possible lines of research, he submitted with good grace to the flat rejection of his proposals, as by Welch's friend Salomonsen. Yet Cohnheim, like most heads of scientific institutes in Germany, required that the work done in his laboratory bear on some large general problem or problems of his own choosing.

Cohnheim, like Ludwig and von Recklinghausen, had learned the first and last secret of teaching creativity in science — almost *not* to teach and never to force. It was, however, no part of their function to give a disinterested and balanced view of the living issues in medical science. Men who were bursting the bounds of the scientific consensus by fresh researches could not be disinterested and for the sake of their advanced students must not be if they could. What they distinctively had to offer was want of balance, one-sidedness, overawareness of the issues dividing them from their rivals, and emotional as well as intellectual involvement in the outcome; all of these contained within the limits of sanity, accompanied by a gift for cutting irretrievable losses in debate, and nicely adapted to the historical situation in pathology. An enormously fruitful sense of tensions and radical antinomies was borne in upon the major figures in the shaping of the pathological tradition.

In many ways the decisive event for the history of pathology in the nineteenth century was the proclamation by Rudolf Virchow of his great dictum that every cell came from another cell. The cell theory supplied the ultimate generalization upon which biology and scientific medicine were henceforth to rest. For the future no explanation of disease could escape the challenge of the microscope and the correlation of functional disorders with structural.

At the other extreme of the middle region where discussions of function and structure blend, François Magendie of Paris was founding in the first half of the century the discipline of experimental physiology, which opened out from another side the possibility of putting theories of disease to the test.

Of the two principal successors of Magendie, his own pupil Claude Bernard and the German Carl Ludwig, Welch wrote home from Leipzig that Bernard was the "more brilliant genius," but that Ludwig surpassed him in "exactness and really scientific investigation." If, in fact, the idea of a "really scientific investigation" did not comprehend for Welch the discovery by Bernard of the storage of sugar in the liver, the role of nerves in regulating the size of blood vessels, and the significance of the pancreatic juice, the fault lay not with Bernard but Welch. But, as Welch implied, Ludwig could never have risen to Bernard's magisterial conception of the "internal environment" within the body which by its stability preserves the life of the organism under stress; and Bernard would never have thought to introduce the improved device for measuring the blood pressure which made Ludwig famous.

The tradition of Magendie came under withering attack from Ludwig's own master, Johannes Müller of Berlin. "How many physiologists," Müller wrote, "expressed their eagerness to make of physiology an experimental science by an aimless cutting open and torturing of a great many animals, of which the results were so often trifling and imperfect." Virchow, the greatest of Müller's pupils, thought of himself as emancipated from this prejudice. But his reputation and his great achievements were those of a pathological anatomist. Of his two most celebrated students, he was therefore closer to von Recklinghausen, an orthodox anatomist of great distinction, than to Cohnheim. The latter had come to be regarded by Welch's time as holding a broader conception of pathology than Virchow and was undoubtedly more of an experimental pathologist — "almost the founder," as Welch wrote to his father in 1877, "and certainly the chief representative of the so-called experimental or physiological school of pathology" with its commitment to the study of "diseased processes induced artificially on animals."

Partly because Virchow had touched and transformed everything, and supplied the canonical point of departure, and partly from some inner necessity of lashing out at one of the two or three great father-figures of the laboratory tradition in Germany, younger men were constrained to make their names by instituting revisions of his thought within the limits set by himself. Thus Cohnheim and his assistant Carl Weigert enjoyed the triumph of overturning Virchow on almost the central problem for pathology, of the nature of inflammation. Virchow had written his inaugural dissertation on the inflamed state of the cornea, a region without blood or lymph vessels, and had been led to depreciate the role of the circulation in producing inflammation. He rightly identified the pus corpuscles associated with inflammation with the leucocytes, or colorless wandering cells found in various circumstances and in various parts of the body; but he denied that the blood was the source of leucocytes. Cohnheim in a famous experiment with the mesentery of a frog actually observed a leucocyte — white corpuscle — passing through the wall of a blood vessel and laid down his celebrated formula "without vessels, no inflammation." The cornea remained lacking in vessels and yet susceptible to something like inflammation, but the tide of opinion set very rapidly against Virchow's conception of a nutritive rather than a circulatory derangement. In another direction, Virchow had assigned a major role in inflammation to the proliferation of cells under the stimulus of irritants. Carl Weigert established the opposite position that irritants led not to cell growth but cell death, so that the fundamental problem was not an excess of vitality but a deficiency. By these bold strokes Cohnheim and Weigert won their independence of the master and set up as his rivals.

Both Cohnheim and Virchow were cast into the shade by the last of the really decisive developments in the history of nineteenth century pathology: the creation of a science of bacteriology by Robert Koch, the man from nowhere. Koch published in 1876 his brilliant researches on the anthrax bacillus, which among other things opened out new vistas of usefulness for botany. In the same year he visited Breslau to demonstrate his anthrax experiments for the great botanist Ferdinand Cohn, who lived and worked in close association with Cohnheim. Cohnheim and Weigert witnessed the demonstration. Koch returned to Breslau in June of 1877, when Cohnheim introduced him to Welch and spoke with enthusiasm of what the visitor had shown and told him.

In spite of this, Welch's friend Salomonsen, a pioneer of bacteriology, was told in the summer of 1877: "You know, the professor doesn't much like people to work with such virulent things in the laboratory." In point of fact, no bacteriological researches were going forward under Cohnheim in Welch's and Salomonsen's time in Breslau. But Weigert's cousin, the handsome blond boy Paul Ehrlich, then twenty-two, was already the true "master dyer" — "always running around among us with blue, yellow, red and green fingers" — and wrists — and preparing to be the founder of the chemotherapy of bacterial disease.

For Welch almost the whole of this situation was transformed from a flat terrain of inert facts, scientific and historical, into a personal experience with the power to etch controversies into relief by the emotional and human tone with which they had been invested for him by mere contact with his teachers. The tone was then deepened by the work which he did under their guidance.

Ludwig passed on to his students a strong preference for "facts" over "theories," the insistence — only natural in a man celebrated for innovations in physiological apparatus — on closer ties between medicine and physics, and above all the suggestion that cellular pathology in the Virchowian tradition ought not to be regarded as the whole science of disease. At least partly on this account, Ludwig and his assistant Hugo Kronecker undertook to divert Welch from Virchow — with whom he had originally planned to study — to the rising star of a more catholic pathology, Julius Cohnheim. With this preference in Ludwig's mind for Cohnheim must have gone the sense that in any event Virchow had now largely retreated into anthropology and politics — he invented the term *Kulturkampf* — and had lost his claim to be in the forefront of the creative thrust in pathology.

It was part of the audacity of the effort to manufacture creative intellects in science that the nineteenth century had an almost paralyzing awareness that creativity and the gift of calling forth creativity in others came and went by no laws. One necessity of the situation therefore became to divert promising students away from the master who was burned out toward the new master who was coming up. The stream of the potentially creative had to be turned at the last moment but not too late. The one conspicuous gap, therefore, in the circle of Welch's teachers in Germany was the result of an affirmative gesture of confidence in the greater vitality of Cohnheim than Virchow and the greater urgency of Cohnheim's researches. Welch was one of the earliest non-German students to study with Cohnheim, and both by being a foreigner and having come from Ludwig, he set the final seal upon Cohnheim's claim to be a master. In this way Welch allowed Ludwig to perform one of the decisive political acts of the scientific community: to give to some of one's colleagues and withhold from others a flow of students of the first rank by whom the participants in the creative tradition might prolong their own

THE CREATIVE TRADITION 47

researches and transmit their ideals and commitments to the future.

The exercise of power, the deflecting of the stream, was accomplished, and Welch went to Cohnheim. From Cohnheim he got two things chiefly: in the first place, an emphasis on the active role of the investigator in inducing pathological states in the animal subject and on the dynamic process by which the anatomical lesions of Virchowian discourse came into being; and in the second place, an absence of really imperious pressures toward an absorption in bacteriology, a not quite sufficient alerting of Welch to the possibilities of the new field. A sense of balance, between cellular pathology and physiological pathology, precisely defined the special contribution of Cohnheim to the shaping of his students' outlook. But the same balance deprived his students of the temporary overemphasis on bacteriology which may well have been a psychological imperative if pathologists were to make adequate room for a new kind of investigation. Cohnheim had indeed made a generous acknowledgment at an early date of the brilliance and skill of Koch's work, and had introduced Welch to Koch. Moreover, the Breslau group included three significant pioneers in bacteriology: Ferdinand Cohn, Carl Weigert, and Welch's own best friend Carl Salomonsen. Yet the whole subject of bacteriology seems to have made no great impression upon him at the time. Though Cohnheim spoke favorably of Koch, he did not give his assent to the new development in the one really persuasive form of rethinking and reshaping the activities of his own institute. Cohnheim did not raise the pressure of his commendation to the threshold of awareness of a student like Welch, still absorbed in digesting the innovations of Cohnheim himself. Welch had undoubtedly set the threshold much too high.

The ultimate sanction in Welch's eyes was necessarily the kind of research enterprise which his teachers allowed him to pursue. He appears to have been entirely passive in this matter. The fact that Welch invariably took up the first suggestion made to him from above was a danger signal, of the docility, receptivity, and want of spontaneity that were death to the creative tradition. But in the treatment of other men's themes Welch reasserted his independence.

The least important of his researches as a student was the first, an investigation of lymphosarcoma — a cancerous condition of the lymph glands — proposed by the pathological anatomist Ernst Wagner of Leipzig. Wagner expressed satisfaction with the results, essentially of a descriptive character, and urged Welch to work them up into an article. Welch soon came to regard this kind of work as the dry husks of the Virchowian tradition in its decline, and never published the article. But he learned from Wagner how to prepare and mount specimens.

Carl Ludwig, a physiologist, set for Welch a problem well within the bounds of classical anatomy: "the microscopical study of the nerves and ganglion cells of the heart." Ludwig had already treated the subject himself a generation earlier, but he told Welch that "new and improved methods," like the impregnation of the finest nerve fibers with gold chloride in the manner of Julius Cohnheim, held out the possibility of fresh discoveries. This work taught Welch how to handle fresh tissues, where his previous work had dealt for the most part with specimens hardened in alcohol. Apart from the mastery of new techniques,

THE CREATIVE TRADITION

Welch's investigation led to a discovery of some importance, "namely that the processes of many of the ganglion cells instead of continuing as independent nerve fibres lose themselves in other nerve fibres forming a T-shaped connection." Welch never published his findings, and the same discovery was made and claimed by Louis-Antoine Ranvier.

When, on the completion of this research, Welch allowed himself to be diverted in the late spring of 1877 from Virchow to Cohnheim, Cohnheim was directing the work of his institute to the problem of edema, the excessive loss of the fluid portions of the blood to the surrounding tissues, with swelling. He had reached the tentative conclusion that edema of the lungs was not the result of blood congestion — imperfect or sluggish flushing of blood from the pulmonary region — a view which if borne out would make pulmonary edema different from edema elsewhere. The subject had not been studied since René Laënnec, of the stethoscope (in 1819), and never experimented upon. Cohnheim turned the whole problem over to Welch — an important theme with historical echoes of great resonance.

Welch began by attempting to produce the condition in animals by obstructing the outflow of blood from the pulmonary vein (leading from the lungs to the left ventricle of the heart) and alternatively from the aorta (the great artery leading away from the left ventricle). He found that edema of the lungs could be produced in this way, but only by an almost total obstruction of the blood current. As the condition was known to exist in human beings who went on living, this explanation would not do. The obvious inference would have been that congestion played no part and that Cohnheim was right; and Welch might have brought his research to the honorable conclusion of having confirmed by ingenious experiments what the best authorities already suspected. But Welch's particular strength as an investigator, his own special gift for recalcitrance in the face of authority, lay in finding what he was expected to find, but stopping to recall that the expected interpretation did not necessarily follow from the expected result. This feeling for the multitude of conflicting hypotheses which could accommodate one and the same empirical fact now came to Welch's aid. He therefore asked if he had exhausted in point of logic the possibilities for producing edema through congestion. "Is it possible to think of anything else which will permit more blood to flow into the lungs than can flow out? It occurred to me that if the left ventricle were paralyzed and the right ventricle still retained its power, the latter could continue to pump blood into the lungs while the former had not strength to pump it out."

The problem remained of putting his hypothesis to the test. He found that heart poisons tended to act equally on both ventricles, and had to adopt "the coarse procedure" of opening the chest in dogs and rabbits and squeezing the left ventricle between his fingers. "Under these circumstances well-marked pulmonary oedema resulted." Cohnheim was greatly impressed by Welch's findings, running counter as they did to his own theories, and encouraged Welch to prepare an article in German for *Virchows Archiv*—"Zur Pathologie des Lungenödems," published in 1878. With this publication, in the best journal of its kind in the world, Welch had entered fully into the community of productive scientists.

Between the first sketch of his ideas and the published article, he introduced a qualification of great interest. He had spoken at first in terms of paralysis of the left ventricle. In the article he took pains to speak instead of a "disproportion *[Missverhältnis]* between the working power of the left ventricle and of the right ventricle of such character that, the resistance remaining the same, the left heart is unable to expel in a unit of time the same quantity of blood as the right heart." Both explicitly and implicitly the formulation had been broadened — and rendered more defensible under attack. Certain critics soon protested that the clinical indications in pulmonary edema ruled out a total paralysis of the left ventricle; and others, including Cohnheim, pointed out that spasm of the ventricle might produce the same result as paralysis. But though Welch's experiments dealt with paralysis, and paralysis only, in generalizing from them he spoke merely of a "disproportion" and so left room for the effect both of spasm and of degrees of enfeeblement short of paralysis. He was therefore able to say that his theory did not exclude the strong pulse detected by his critics.

The beginner who had not been fit for von Recklinghausen's laboratory two years before now returned to Strassburg with technique, insights, and a style of his own in research. Von Recklinghausen, the opposite pole to Cohnheim among the students of Virchow, seized the opportunity to confront Welch with the chief issue between Cohnheim and Virchow — whether the pus bodies were or were not identical with the white corpuscles of the blood. Cohnheim had proved that in some instances they were, and the conviction was widespread that they always were. But Virchow had begun his career by studying the puslike formations in the cornea, a region without blood or lymph vessels, and the decision had only gone to Cohnheim by one of the recurring acts of faith familiar in the history of science, that some "facts" will prove to be anomalies that have to be cleared away, and others, of the same apparent standing, will survive and gather confirmation to themselves.

Von Recklinghausen now proposed that Welch return to the historic problem of inflammation of the cornea, for the second time to renew the researches of one of the legendary figures in pathology. Welch confirmed Virchow's original findings, but then exercised his gift for avoiding the obvious (but mistaken) interpretation of his own work. The cells which he saw proceeding to the site of irritation in a cornea could not be white corpuscles and looked like pus; but he refused to conclude what von Recklinghausen would have been glad to hear, that pus arises not from white corpuscles but from fixed tissue cells. Here Welch was justified by the event — the puslike substance of the inflamed cornea was later shown not to be pus. The personal relationship to Virchow that Ludwig had induced Welch to forego was not to be made good by joining in Virchow's errors at the behest of von Recklinghausen. With this scientifically inconclusive, but in human and psychological terms quite conclusive, research, Welch ended his stay in Europe where he had begun, in Strassburg.

Welch was a man of the laboratory, but also a man; and the laboratories were a world of their own, but also Germany. His initiation into the creative life was therefore an initiation also into life abroad and a first opportunity to see America in perspective. Many things in Germany he did not like — the heavy food, cooked to death; the "reckless" members of the student corps with their foolish little caps and their dueling scars; the academic wives, with no tact or conversation, and almost always "inferior to the husband"; and the great army of German chauvinists, arrogant to the bone and swollen with contempt for the rest of the world since the Franco-Prussian War. His own teacher Ernst Wagner had told him with overbearing assurance that America would yet have a king.

Welch never mixed very freely with the ordinary German students, or the German public, but he came to be extremely fond of his teachers and fellow research workers in their native milieu: the group in Leipzig joining to give Welch and three others who were going away an evening of songs, toasts, and mock poetry; Weigert's friends putting garlands on his microscope and chair and printing WELCOME on the window with aniline dyes; "Prof. Waldeyer, with whom I study microscopy" coming to drink a beer to the health of his American student "as if we were life long friends"; the botanical society of Breslau climbing a mountain, followed by a band playing music, through meadows and groves full of wild flowers till they reached a ruin at the top and looked out across the valley — "in the distance the Schneekoppe, clad with snow, and the more modest peaks of the same mountain chain, around us the hillsides with pine and chestnut groves, at our feet the quiet valley and gay meadows." The great Ferdinand Cohn, the first botanist of his time, repeated to Welch on this occasion the lines of Goethe, "America, you have it better than the Old World — no fallen castles and no basalt stones." But Welch might well have heard this tribute with mixed feelings and wondered to himself if everything was not of a piece — the German *Gemütlichkeit,* the melting haze that lay over the Riesengebirge, the absence as he thought of "haste" and "friction" that left room for botanical excursions (followed by a band), the giant Cohn linking hands with an unbroken line of scholars backward through time, and the whole steeping of European experience in infinite expanses of time which had built castles and let them fall into ruins — and doubted whether he could disengage the laboratory tradition from its native habitat and transplant it to the raw New World with no past and no repose.

The only chance seemed to turn on the fate of the Johns Hopkins University. At the opening ceremonies in 1876, the agnostic Huxley delivered the main address — and no one delivered a prayer. Welch observed the resulting furor from Europe and dispatched a memorandum to his sister Emma. He supposed that the people who were indignant about Huxley would end by agreeing with the president of Drew Seminary that "only ministers of the gospel should be college professors." Welch for his part was "sorry for those whose faith in God can only stand or fall with the truth or falsity of Darwinism, for it seems to me no longer doubtful but that the theory of evolution will prevail." Welch had been converted to evolution partly by attending the Leipzig lectures of Rudolf Leuckart on comparative anatomy; and as he told his father, "That there is anything irreligious about the doctrine I can not see." But while he was in Germany he stopped going to church and returned to the United States with no real commitment to religion; so that he would probably not have cared much if evolution did conflict with religion. Buckle had had the better of Grandma Welch after all. The weight of the Puritan tradition was rolled away forever. About the prospects of the

THE CREATIVE TRADITION 55

Johns Hopkins University Welch did care greatly, and he would tolerate no attack upon it.

The great question that hung over his whole time in Germany was whether someone else might get the appointment, on which his whole future was predicated, as professor of pathology in the Johns Hopkins medical school. While he was still in Leipzig his teacher Wagner had brought into the laboratory a tall stiff man from America, John Shaw Billings, the founder of the Army Medical Library in Washington and now the chief figure in planning for the new medical school. He and Welch went in the evening to Auerbach's Keller, where Faust met the Devil, and talked and drank beer but mostly talked. Billings said that there would be laboratories on the German model, high admission standards, and small classes. In many fields Billings did not consider that any competent man existed in America, and young men would, if necessary, be sent to Germany to fit themselves for professorships. "Of course," Welch wrote home, "such young men would at first be taken on trial and not made full professors."

Billings made a note of Welch's name and address and said that the university would have to look to men like him to fill the chairs. Welch was encouraged but cautious in his expectations. "All these hopes seem very airy and egotistical when I think of the numbers of able young men who have been and are over here, some having acquired already some reputation, and who are hoping for the same or similar prospects."

Above all, Welch was haunted by the specter of a young American of his own age, named T. Mitchell Prudden — a graduate of Yale and the College of Physicians and Surgeons of New York, whom he had not, however, met. "I do not know him," Welch wrote to his friend and self-appointed patron Fred Dennis, "but undoubtedly he will become a swell at pathology and join the army intending to march on the Johns Hopkins. I expect that he is a pet of Gilman's. Did not Gilman mention his name to you?" When Welch got a false report from Dennis in the fall of 1877 that the chair had been filled, he said that if someone of established reputation like Francis Delafield had been chosen, he would not complain; but if it were Prudden he would feel "a little sore." In October of 1877 Welch finally caught up with Prudden in Vienna and managed to do justice to his good qualities. "He is a very good fellow and I think an excellent microscopist and pathologist. I do not think he has anything to look forward to in America more than I have in a pathological line." But a thousand other men, or Prudden himself, might still win the prize, and it was an open question when Welch sailed for home in February 1878 whether he would be any different from the other American students of whom Carl Ludwig said to him that they did brilliant work in Germany but were never heard from again. It remained to be seen whether the creative tradition in science could be made an article of export.

V

New York: the Second Phase

THE AMERICANS who went to Europe before the Civil War had been looking for something to take back with them. Some of the artists and writers of Welch's generation were looking not for objects for the home but for a home to be at home in. The men of science, however, were almost entirely exempt from this new turn in the cultural affairs of the Western world. Yet they had no illusions as to what they were returning to. Of his own interests, Welch wrote immediately after his return that "there is no opportunity for, no appreciation of, no demand for that kind of work here." "I sometimes feel rather blue when I look ahead and see that I am not going to be able to realize my aspirations in life." He could quiz students, teach elementary microscopy and pathology, and build up a consulting practice to support himself — "but that is all patchwork and the drudgery of life and what hundreds do." He thought that he would never be free of these trammels. Two men whom he met in New York had also studied pathology in Germany. One hoped to go back to Europe and stay and the other would go "if he had any idea he could make a living there." "Do not be alarmed," Welch wrote to his sister. "I do not expect to go, but I do think that the condition of medical education here is simply horrible."

The logic of the situation was inescapable but failed to send the men of science back to the more congenial environment of Europe. Perhaps the explanation lay in the fact that the "living" of a scientist required an institutional base as that of the artist did not, and the competition for academic positions in Europe was desperate. Whatever the cause, Welch was the type of the American students of science in Europe in always meaning to go home again — perhaps to the death of the inner life, but home.

In the last days of his stay in Europe, in January 1878, when he was visiting Paris, Welch learned that Fred Dennis had secured for him appointments as demonstrator of pathological anatomy in the summer term at the Bellevue Hospital Medical College and assistant to the great Austin Flint, Sr., leader of the Bellevue school and of the medical profession in New York City. But Welch, who was now accustomed to hearing that Fred Dennis had settled his career for him, declined to commit himself. He was, after all, a graduate of the College of Physicians and Surgeons, and favorably known there, and might hope for a connection with the best rather than the second-best of the New York schools.

He therefore bearded one of the "Brahmins" of Physicians and Surgeons, his former teacher Francis Delafield, and asked for a job. Delafield promptly offered him an unpaid lectureship on pathology in the summer term — the doldrums of the medical year, when young men were given the chance to fill in in responsible positions. Welch replied that he was more interested in giving a laboratory course, and Delafield said that by all means he should —

if he could find a vacant room in the college building. There were no vacant rooms in the college building. There were no vacant rooms in the Y.M.C.A. building across the street. There were no vacant rooms. When the downcast Welch reported his lack of success, Delafield took the issue as settled: all rooms were occupied; no occupants could be displaced; and what the physical plant and the existing allotment of space did not allow for could not be. The offer of a summer lectureship stood, but Welch was not yet prepared to capitulate and turned his back on Physicians and Surgeons. He would have to be Fred Dennis's man after all, and make a career at Bellevue. But he meant this career to be more than Dennis had intended, with the conduct of a laboratory involved in it somewhere.

He therefore stepped down to the level of Bellevue and entered into weeks of tortuous negotiations for setting up a laboratory there. In the end he obtained three rooms and some kitchen tables with nothing on them; no microscopes, no microtomes, no specimens. He later estimated that the authorities at Bellevue had spent "fully twenty-five dollars" on his behalf. They got for their money the first teaching laboratory for pathology in America. If, as subsequently appeared, they thought that they had bought and paid for Welch into the bargain, they gave him the two indispensable things for his work in life: the aura that goes with the luck that is not entirely luck of being not the second or third but the first in any field; and a chance to impose himself in all of his singularity upon the imagination of the young men before their vision was distracted by other people. And, for all of this, there had not been much time; for Prudden, if no one else, was already on the scene and looking for some sort of foothold — the same sort.

The prize was Welch's and his myth now began to take shape — the efforts to say how "Billy" Welch looked, and what he gave forth, and how he drew his students into the center of things and gave them the sense of being borne forward on one of the main historical currents of the nineteenth century. He moved easily among them, "a chubby, round-faced, pink-cheeked, somewhat snub-nosed, quick-moving youngish man," balding, with "small feet and small adroit hands," well dressed in a close-fitting cutaway; helping students to improvise from darning needles or pieces of old wire the teasers necessary for shredding microscopic specimens; rushing off with his class to an optical store which reported a new shipment of slides from Germany; looking gravely at connective tissue from the tail of a rat "as if he had never seen such a specimen"; and escorting frogs for the laboratory from Norfolk by Pullman, to the consternation of the other passengers at the accompanying uproar.

One of the students who came to Welch was a rich young man from Princeton, Henry Fairfield Osborn — "a most promising young man, the best pupil whom I ever had," Welch wrote at the time. Osborn wanted to study under the microscope as many unusual animals as he could, and it fell to Welch to keep the supply coming. He knew of at least one place to turn. His old teacher Seguin had performed one last historic service for Welch by having him to dinner at Delmonico's for a small, olive-complexioned man from Montreal, with a great drooping mustache, the "black Celt" William Osler. Osler, not yet thirty, was the first medical man who had really taken in the fact of the railroads as a means to professional success and usefulness. By the time that Welch met him in New York, Osler had already begun to make the train routes a kind of private resource for getting himself known all over eastern Canada and the United States — dropping in on the physicians of one city after another, opening up a new professional terrain and a new sphere of influence each time, a rail-borne liaison man and a unifying and pacificatory force in the medical profession of a whole continent. He "captivated" Welch, and it seemed a natural thing to see if he would ship Canadian fauna to Henry Fairfield Osborn. He would and did, and the relationship with Welch was cemented.

After Welch had launched his laboratory successfully, the College of Physicians and Surgeons had to bestir itself, and early in the fall of 1878 Delafield informed him that the alumni had contributed the necessary funds for building a laboratory in histology and pathology. The college building still contained the same number of fully occupied rooms; but the ice-cream parlor on the ground floor would simply have to go. Delafield himself was to be in general charge, with Welch as his first assistant and head of the work in histology, at $500 a year for the first year with more thereafter.

He could now have what he had always wanted, a connection with the College of Physicians and Surgeons, with the additional inducement of a new rule requiring all students to work in the laboratory as well as the dissecting room. Welch was delighted and saw no reason why he should not accept — until he talked with the men at Bellevue, who represented it as not quite "the square thing" to leave. In this atmosphere of mutterings about treason and bad faith he felt obliged to refuse Delafield's offer. Delafield responded by asking him to suggest someone else; and Welch had to put forward for the post which he himself would have liked to have, his old rival T. Mitchell Prudden, a lean retiring young man with a disproportionate mustache and not much juice in his personality, but an able pathologist and now a good friend of Welch. "I feel," Welch wrote to Prudden, "as if I were relinquishing a great opportunity and do not see any equivalent for it at present at Bellevue."

In addition to his central task of establishing a laboratory tradition in pathology, Welch was busy with many other things. He shared with Fred Dennis the post of demonstrator of anatomy at Bellevue and once a week performed an autopsy "à la Welch" before the class with "free swooping strokes." From the beginning he also lectured on pathology in the summer; but not until 1882–1883, when he had been at Bellevue for four years, was he allowed to lecture in the winter term.

His lectures began with a warning that he would not give the detailed synoptic view of his subject as was customary, and that he would sooner show the student something than tell them about it. "Didactic instruction" they could get from books, but pathological histology could "only be learned by practical work with the microscope in a laboratory." His lectures were different in tone as well as content, clear and lucid rather than rhetorical.

Still another of Welch's roles was that of assistant to Austin Flint, Sr., one of the appointments prearranged by Dennis. Flint, with his minuscule spectacles and billowing mutton-chop whiskers — a made man but not petrified — was the author of the standard American *Principles and Practice of Medicine* (first edition, 1866). For the edition of 1881 he enlisted the help of Welch on pathology and so assimilated the work of the Germans to his own.

The least congenial of all Welch's activities — apart from a halfhearted effort to get started in private practice — was participation in a "quiz" with Dr. Henry Goldthwaite. Close instruction in comparatively small groups, with opportunity for recitation, could not be had within the formal structure of the medical schools. As a result extramural quizzes sprang up, normally conducted by teachers in the various medical schools and devoted to preparing men to pass the written examinations for their degrees and, more important, the examinations for internships and commissions in the army and navy. The going rate for the better quizzes was $100 per student, everything included; and Welch and Goldthwaite did a thriving business at this price. But the commodity in which the quizzes dealt was not insight or understanding but negotiable and producible information; and Welch withdrew with a sense of relief at the earliest possible moment. For once, however, his imagination had flagged; he had failed to see what might be done even with the contemptible quiz.

Soon after his return from Europe, early in 1878, Welch had met one of the long line of Yale men who had gone on to Physicians and Surgeons, a tall, slim, balding fellow with the ears of a satyr, named William S. Halsted. In New Haven, Halsted had been a crew man and captain of the football team, and a poor student who never charged a book out of the Yale library. But in New York he had taken a serious interest in surgery, and in 1878 went abroad to study under the great German surgeons. He returned to America in 1880, still the outgoing animal man of his days at Yale — "a model," in Welch's words, "of muscular strength and vigor, full of enthusiasm and of the joy of life." Welch and many other congenial bachelors fell into the habit of dining regularly at the big house kept up by Halsted and a doctor friend of his. To Welch, Halsted was the symbol of an overflowing gusto, verve, and dash that he himself could never attain.

In the medical profession of New York, Halsted, with his qualities of "brilliancy, boldness and manual dexterity," shot upward like a rocket. In addition to making his reputation as a surgeon, he organized a dispensary at the Roosevelt Hospital and made of it "a lively center for the study of injuries and diseases in ambulatory patients," the first experiment of its kind in the city. But Halsted's force of will and intellectual grasp were even better demonstrated in the transformation which he effected in the old institution of the quiz. He sent his quiz men to the dispensary and also to Welch's laboratory at Bellevue, worked with dry and wet specimens in teaching anatomy, and — like Welch in his lectures at Bellevue — failed to give the even-handed review of materials to be learned by rote, which had always been the substance of lectures and quizzes alike. He made of the quiz something different — the bringing together of a new kind of faculty with a new curriculum and new methods of teaching.

On his return to New York, Welch had written of the existing medical schools that they were "simply horrible." But he, Prudden, and Halsted successfully instituted a movement to which little attention has been paid as a cooperative and almost a corporate enterprise: a reform of the old system of medical education partly from within, so that a self-cure, of an agonizing slowness, of the proprietary schools may be said to have begun in New York and partly by reason of the very defects of the system. The weakness of the existing schools helped the three men to build, within a surprisingly short time, a kind of medical faculty of their own, cutting across institutional lines, silently eluding the seniority system — of a Congressional inflexibility — of the medical professors, and giving beneath the surface and in the interstices of the formal instruction an almost Germanic tutelage — a shadow medical college of the city of New York uniting the best resources of all the schools.

Welch might well have taken satisfaction in what he had done to raise the level of medical instruction in New York. His own laboratory at Bellevue had to be enlarged in 1882 to accommodate the growing numbers of students. But at the one decisive point he had failed to keep the faith with von Recklinghausen, Cohnheim, and Ludwig. He had given no evidence of being a self-winding participant in the creative tradition. In his period in New York he carried through to completion only one piece of investigation, and this in collaboration with and at the suggestion of another man, the distinguished physiologist Samuel J. Meltzer. They shook up red blood corpuscles with abrasive particles and demonstrated that by this mechanical process the corpuscles as such could be made to disappear in their entirety. The research was not of great importance, and the impulse behind it had come from someone else. Welch was a man with almost no capacity for self-deception, and he saw clearly that by his own standards he had made no success at all.

As always, the way out could only be Johns Hopkins. With every successive step since 1876 Welch's first ambition had sharpened and defined itself into the one absolute necessity of his life. By 1884 Billings and Gilman were finally prepared to act, and Billings went to New York at the end of February to refresh his impressions of Welch. Gilman had written for advice to the great physiologist Willy Kühne, the pioneer of enzyme research, who recommended Welch and a young Englishman. Kühne added, however, that the man really to be consulted was Julius Cohnheim. When, therefore, Billings went to New York, Cohnheim had already written to Gilman that "the person best fitted for the chair of general pathology is Mr. Welch of New York. Welch worked with me for a long time and I regard him as an acute as well as a thoughtful investigator." Cohnheim died in August of the same year, at the age of forty-five, and Welch later heard from his widow that he had dictated the letter to Gilman while "very ill and suffering greatly." Thus at a time when Welch must have been profoundly depressed by the thought of having let his teachers in Germany down, Cohnheim was making one last gesture of confidence in him.

On March 1, Billings wrote to Gilman to sum up his estimate of Welch, then thirty-three — "modest, quiet, and a gentleman in every sense," "a good lecturer," and "an excellent laboratory teacher" with "a keen desire for an opportunity to make original investigations." "He has been trying to make some original investigations in the causes and pathology of Dysentery but has very little time as he has to make his living by students and Doctors fees and must give them the first place." Billings concluded "upon the whole" that Welch was "the best man in this country for the Hopkins."

Gilman therefore asked Welch to come to Baltimore, to meet himself, two of the trustees, and the two members of the Philosophical Faculty of the University who were expected to help in laying the scientific foundations of the medical school, the chemist Ira Remsen and the biologist H. Newell Martin. The interview went off well in spite of the fact that because of an injured heel Welch's footwear did not match. "Wait a moment, Dr. Welch," Gilman had said. "The Johns Hopkins does not regard eccentricity as a sign of intelligence."

On March 15, Gilman wrote to Welch asking permission to place his name before the trustees as professor of pathology. The salary was to be $4000 for the first two years, $4500 for the next two, and then $5000. "It is expected that you will have such laboratory facilities and assistants as may be requisite." With the formal offer of the chair, Gilman enclosed a personal note to say that the action was "hearty, unanimous and earnest. . . . *You must come.*" His was to be the first appointment to the medical faculty, and, as he knew from his visit to Baltimore, he would be expected to play a leading role — with Billings, Remsen, and Martin — in making the policies of the medical school and choosing the other professors.

Now that the great opportunity had come, it became a matter of genuine doubt whether Welch would accept. His impulses toward research, the whole history of his education of himself, his distaste for the "drudgery" of routine teaching, all pointed toward acceptance: "My inclinations," he wrote to Gilman, "are most decidedly toward accepting the position." But his friends in New York conspired to give to the fulfillment of his ambitions a bitter taste. Welch had said that he "dreaded" his interview with Dennis, and he had not shared quarters with Dennis for two years without learning to know his character.

Dennis refused to hear of Welch's going and set to work to make it impossible. Welch felt that he was bound to state certain conditions which, if met, would induce him to stay in New York: he must have an adequate laboratory, with an endowed salary of $4000 for himself and $1000 for an assistant. When Dennis got Andrew Carnegie to pledge $50,000 for a separate research laboratory in pathology at Bellevue, and the trustees of Bellevue appropriated $45,000 for the purchase of a site, he thought that he had brought Welch back under control. He tried to bring additional pressure to bear through the members of Welch's own family. Dennis wrote to Welch's brother-in-law that the choice was between an income of $20,000 as "the leading man in New York and hence in America" and $10,000 as "a scientific recluse" in a "provincial city among untried and inexperienced persons." "His ideas imbibed in Germany are impractical in our form of government. He must cut himself aloof from everything in the way of sacred associations and of true friendships and of worldly emoluments for an ideal, which can not ever be realized." Dennis succeeded in bringing old William Wickham Welch into camp — but not the tough-minded stepmother, whom Welch now knew to be the most understanding of his relatives.

Dennis chose to claim that he had met the conditions laid down by Welch, but his idea of meeting the requirement that the salary of two men be endowed was to say that Welch could make enough money from consulting and student fees to carry the salaries himself. Welch therefore accepted the chair at Johns Hopkins at the end of March. In his own mind he had held from beginning to end to what he had written to his father on returning from Johns Hopkins: "My energies are split up in too many directions and are likely to be so long as I remain here." In Baltimore, everything would be "quieter, more academic," and he could give himself up to "original work." The Hopkins geologist George H. Williams had spoken for Welch himself: ". . . it is an opportunity for giving a start and impetus to the spirit of real scientific work which is thus far so sadly lacking on this side of the Atlantic, which can come to a man only once in a lifetime."

Welch, who had found Dennis self-indulgent and immoderate in doing favors, now found him self-indulgent and intemperate in venting spleen. But in one sense Dennis by his very extravagance destroyed the effect he was aiming at. Welch saw clearly for the first time that to save himself whole and be his own man he had had at any cost to go away from New York. He now began to think of the call to Baltimore in the new light of "a deliverance from oppressive and compromising environments." As he wrote to his stepmother, "It looks almost as if Dr. Dennis thought that he had a lien upon my whole future life." For his part, he regretted that "a life-long friendship should thus come to an end," but he had nothing to reproach himself for.

Though Dennis's attitude showed that it was necessary for Welch to go and go at once, the episode left a deep scar. Welch never again trusted a man as he had trusted Dennis, or put himself for good or evil in the same way in another man's power. From this time forward all men seemed to know Welch well from their first meeting — and almost never knew him better. The only freedom that seemed to lie open to him in his private life was to avoid all ties of intimacy: first with women, and then with men. The less constricted but more perilous freedom of the deeply engaged, he was cut off from through the whole of his mature life.

Though the decision to go to Baltimore involved an emotional impoverishment of the private man, it enlarged his professional potentialities in a way not possible in New York. No one city could be allowed to monopolize the tradition of scientific medicine, if the Americans were to avoid the mistakes of the French; and the fact of his going while under such pressures to stay was a symbol that cultural sovereignty was to be dispersed beyond repair. That Baltimore had been until recently one of the most apathetic of the large cities intellectually merely heightened the effect. But if not to Baltimore, Welch would have had to go somewhere other than Boston, New York, or Philadelphia, to fulfill his role in history and be the maker of something altogether new and not the mender and patcher of something old. He was and had to be for his maximum usefulness a doctrinaire — an affable doctrinaire with the art of biding his time, but a doctrinaire unafraid of clean starts and symbolic gestures of defiance.

VI
The Last Student Days

IN THE INTERVAL between his return from Germany in 1878 and his appointment to the faculty of Johns Hopkins in 1884, Welch found himself trapped by the quickening tempo of science. Cohnheim had told him forcefully of the significance of Koch's work in bacteriology, and Welch had neglected the hint; but within a few years to study bacteriology had become an imperative. Welch had therefore found himself, immediately on the completion of his studies, under the best men in the best universities, the representative of a dying epoch in the history of pathology — the short but decisive epoch of Cohnheim, which had followed on the long supremacy of Virchow and had now been succeeded by the age of bacteriology. Welch had thought that he was moving with the stream of history, but the stream had been diverted and unless he agreed to be left behind he would have to re-enter the stream where it allowed of entry and flow in the new direction.

Welch in New York had followed the new developments sympathetically, and in this had the encouragement of his chief, the elder Flint, who was an enthusiastic "bacterian" at a time when men of his age and standing in America tended to be either skeptical or hostile. One morning in

1882 Flint came bounding up the stairs in Welch's house, waving a newspaper and crying to the dazed Welch, still in bed sleeping off a late night in the dead house, "I knew it, I knew it!" Koch's great discovery of the tubercle bacillus had been announced in the papers.

Shortly thereafter Welch demonstrated the discovery before his laboratory class at Bellevue. One of the students, a dark young man with hair *en brosse* and a large mustache, never forgot the occasion. "He showed us methods of staining sputum and demonstrating the tubercle bacillus. I can now see quite clearly the steam rising from the dish of carbol-fuchsin in the sand-bath containing the sputum while he talked." The student's name was Hermann M. Biggs, and from this first inspiration he went on to become a bacteriologist and the leader of the public health movement in America. To the end of his life when some innovation appeared, Biggs would ask, "What does Welch think of it?"

In 1882 men wanted to know what the leaders of the profession in New York thought, as the talk went around of what Welch had done in his laboratory. The celebrated diagnostician Alfred L. Loomis of New York University gave his judgment by peering humorously about him and saying to applause, "People say there are bacteria in the air, but I cannot see them." On this Welch passed judgment in turn: "That's too bad. Loomis is such a nice man."

By the standards of New York, Welch had taken the lead in bacteriology, but in fact he lacked the apparatus for original researches and also the perfection of technique needed for establishing in any given instance that bacteria were not, as the better-informed critics of bacteriology claimed, mere concomitants or end products of disease, but the true causative agents. Welch later wrote that he was glad that he had not been able to take up bacteriology at this time, for he would probably have fallen into grave errors and made "a melancholy failure." The only recourse was to go back to Germany and if possible to study with Robert Koch himself. After drawing up at Gilman's request a plan for the new department of pathology in Baltimore, Welch therefore set sail in September 1884. He found on board ship a letter from Fred Dennis telling him to consider their friendship at an end. On his first trip to Europe, Dennis's father had met the passage.

Welch hurried to Berlin to see Koch, who had now retreated behind a forest of beard and left only his troubled sharp eyes naked to the world — Koch the discoverer of the anthrax and tubercle bacilli, and the emissary who had just been sent to India and Egypt to treat with the enemy advancing on Europe from the East, the dreaded Asiatic cholera. Welch was kindly received but told that for the present Koch could not accept him as a student.

Following Koch's advice, he enrolled in November 1884 in the course given in Munich by Koch's own student Wilhelm Frobenius. Welch found this, the first public course in bacteriology ever given anywhere in the world, adequate in its coverage but weighed down by the determination to instill every word and even motion of Koch. In Munich, Welch also found Max von Pettenkofer, the founder of the laboratory tradition in hygiene. Pettenkofer not unnaturally emphasized the role of the physical environment in health and sickness and took as an affront to the whole hygienic tradition which he had created, a germ theory which narrowed the effectual environment of disease to the particular form of specific microorganisms. The idea that

Welch took away with him from this first contact with Pettenkofer and never forgot was the possibility of a laboratory tradition in hygiene and public health.

At the beginning of 1885 Welch moved on by way of Vienna, Budapest, and Prague to Leipzig and Carl Ludwig. Carl Weigert was also in Leipzig — forty years old, not yet a professor, and heartbroken at not being nominated to succeed Cohnheim. One terrible derogation from the atmosphere of freedom for the creative linked the German laboratory tradition of the nineteenth century with the world of total unfreedom that the whole German people built for themselves in the twentieth. Cohnheim was an academic Jew, who succeeded in being treated — almost — as if he were not. Weigert was an academic Jew.

As Welch waited for an opportunity to work with Koch in Berlin, he carried out an inconclusive piece of research under Carl Ludwig. Much as he valued the opportunity for contact with Ludwig, Welch was growing more and more impatient to get on with the study of bacteriology; and he spent the spring vacation period at Leipzig working under the bacteriologist Karl Flügge at Göttingen. In May he went to England to buy physiological instruments for Johns Hopkins and returned to Germany by way of Paris, but did not stop off. "There is nothing especial of a scientific nature to lead me there." Pasteur was then at work in Paris.

In July 1885 the time at last came when Welch could begin a month's laboratory course under Robert Koch. One of the other students was T. Mitchell Prudden. Having studied with both Frobenius and Flügge, Welch found much of the work in Berlin repetitious — but also "very interesting and profitable." The key to the paradox may be found in what he always told young men in later years as they departed for Europe. "You must get into contact with the great teachers. Then you will have an impression of the men and their work which you will never forget, and every time you read their writings you will remember. Everything will be much more vivid to you."

Welch found Koch "in every way most approachable and affable — indeed in those days he was one of the most simple-minded, unaffected men imaginable." From time to time he would join Welch and the other students at a restaurant and drink beer with them, never talkative but able to tell a story with "dry wit and humor." But though Welch found Koch to be what some people thought he shortly ceased to be (or doubted that he had ever been), approachable, kindly, and unsuspicious, there was a deep fund of reserve in Koch, heightened by a strong sense of the equivocal bearing of the science which he had brought into being. For Koch perceived that bacteriology was entirely neutral and might be a force either for good or for evil. When he isolated the comma bacillus in Egypt and India, he deliberately destroyed his supply before returning to Europe; and the cultures which he later obtained on the outbreak of cholera in France were kept in the most secure place in his laboratory and handled only by himself.

Both Welch and Prudden were collecting cultures to take back to America, and had acquired from other sources the deadly cholera bacillus. One evening Koch remarked to them, ". . . it would be better a man had never been born if he introduced a disease germ into a region where it previously had not existed — suppose they escaped — suppose it could be traced to an accident in the laboratory —

better that man had never been born!" Welch could not sleep for thinking of this warning. At dawn he took his culture of living cholera bacilli from its secret place and hurried down to the Spree to put the unclean stuff from him. As he was about to throw the tube from a bridge, a furtive-looking figure came scurrying through the empty streets toward the spot. Welch froze in his place. It was his friend Prudden, on the same mission. They jointly threw their tubes in the water, and together saw with horrified fascination that the tubes did not sink but floated serenely down stream. As Welch pointed out, the cholera did not come to Berlin for some little time.

He had now made good the deficiency in his training and was no longer in danger of ranking as one of the last figures of the previous epoch in the history of pathology. He had drawn abreast of the present, and he sailed for home and the future in August 1885. In the fall he took up his duties in Baltimore.

VII
The Johns Hopkins Hospital

BALTIMORE in the 1880's was much the city that it had been twenty years before or would be twenty but not twenty-five years later: "repeated vistas of little brick-faced and protrusively door-stepped houses," always three steps and no more, and white, with shade trees everywhere; Southern "with no southern looseness," but almost Mediterranean in the way that the people lived toward the backs of the houses and in the back yards and gardens and let the omens of their private lives be read in the floods that ran in the open gutters and lapped at the corner steppingstones — bluing water on Monday, soapy water on Saturday night, and raw sewage all the time; dirty with open privies and fly-ridden milk delivered in great uncovered cans, and typhoid drinking water; three distinctive ways of life compacted but not mingled together: for the white people of family, the Monday germans and Madeira and terrapin and clubs where a man might dance a toe dance on a table at an ushers' dinner and cut himself on a champagne glass and have a distracted friend break a gold-headed cane in two for a splint; for the middle sort of Germans, work and beer with oysters and crabs and music; for the Negro people the opening out of life in the hot summertime "and the summer evenings when they wandered, and the noises in the full streets, and the music of the organs, and the dancing, and the warm smell of the people, and of dogs and of the horses, and all the joy of the strong, sweet, pungent, dirty, moist Negro southern summer," and over all "many simple jokes and always wide abandonment of laughter."

Into this old Baltimore Welch came and made himself at home and found his own characteristic world, so that he seemed almost the least Yankee of all the New Englanders who made their fortunes elsewhere. He took furnished rooms on one of the "good" streets — Cathedral — with the family of an impoverished gentlewoman and moved with her to another good street and let himself be inherited in time by her daughter, joined the Maryland Club with its matchless cuisine and rats behind the wainscoting — the usher's toe dance took place at the Baltimore Club, which was something else again — and firmly resisted all efforts to marry him off to one eligible beauty or another until people gave up the cause as lost.

Though Welch blended with the background and took on a protective coloration of the old Maryland tone, he came as the representative of a new and not altogether welcome element in the life of Baltimore. Before the founding of the Johns Hopkins University in 1876, there had been in Baltimore no institutional base for intellectual activities. Henry James still found at the beginning of the twentieth century no "facts" in Baltimore "of any perceptibly public, any majestic or impressive or competitive order" to obstruct one's view of the university. The rearing up of this one mountain above the plain — as President

Eliot of Harvard later pointed out, not because of any widespread public spirit or civic enterprise, but simply because one man willed it — came as a shock and an occasion for taking offense. In Baltimore, as elsewhere, many people were put off by "Huxley without prayers" at the opening exercises of the university; but the abiding offense went much deeper. There had been an irruption into the placid and undemanding intellectual life of Baltimore of the whole conception of rigorous standards of thought and an intransigent defiance of the second-rate and the locally negotiable. Of this defiance the chief symbol was the canvassing and recruiting of the faculty members from all over the United States and western Europe.

In the original faculty of philosophy, not one man was a Baltimorean or even a Marylander, and two, the great mathematician J. J. Sylvester and the brilliant young physiologist H. Newell Martin, were Englishmen. In "philosophy," however, there had never been any pretense of higher instruction in Baltimore. But in the field of medical instruction, the American tradition was that any place that could be described as either a "gateway" (with two railroad stations) or a "center" (hovering in the neighborhood of 50,000 people) could make up an adequate faculty from among the local physicians. Baltimore was a gateway and a center several times over, a port, and even a metropolis, and had the accompanying perquisite of a number of proprietary medical schools, including most notably "the so-called medical department of the so-called University of Maryland," founded in 1807, and the College of Physicians and Surgeons, founded in 1872. The former had in fact no university connection and no serious pretensions to a university standard, but was secure in history as the fountainhead of a disastrous innovation, the granting of medical degrees *and* the right to practice by a proprietary school with no true academic affiliations. The two leading schools in Baltimore at the time when Welch received his call to Johns Hopkins were far from being the worst in America, and the expectation might have been that a few of the very best of the local practitioners and teachers of medicine would be skimmed off for the new school.

The coming of Welch was a symbol that the local product would not do. The "nationalizing" of the faculties was to be complete and the example set by the Hopkins unequivocal through the whole range of appointments. No other American institution had ever made such root-and-branch warfare on academic provincialism. When to the feeling of hurt and perplexity that this attitude called forth was added the fact that the Johns Hopkins University was endowed beyond any precedent and could pay the medical professors good though not munificent salaries, the misgivings of the local profession were understandable: prominent physicians and consultants like Welch would probably be brought in from the outside and subsidized in their efforts to snatch the most attractive fees from the accustomed local hands. The fact that Welch was well liked in this atmosphere from the outset of his career in Baltimore, and better liked from year to year, undoubtedly arose in part from the circumstance that he never engaged in practice or consultation of any kind. As early as 1891 he was elected president of the state medical society, known by the resounding name of the Medical and Chirurgical Faculty of Maryland. But it was his genius to be well liked without making any concessions in principle, and his presence in Baltimore, however soothing in itself, made certain that the alien university spirit would prevail through all of the foundations created by Johns Hopkins.

In the letter drawn up for the guidance of his trustees, Hopkins had written: "Bear constantly in mind that it is my wish and purpose that the Hospital shall ultimately form a part of the Medical School of that University, for which I have made ample provision by my Will." This injunction made Johns Hopkins almost unique among the great educational philanthropists in giving not only vast sums of money but a philosophy and a tradition on the same scale. The decisive innovation was that of a hospital subordinated to the purposes of a medical school, and both to those of a university, and conversely a university tradition in medicine forced to take account of the resources for medical instruction of a great hospital.

Whether, if the faculty of philosophy and the hospital, let alone the medical school, had come into being at the same time, the ideal of Johns Hopkins could have been realized may be doubted. But in point of fact, the university proper came first, the hospital staff second, the opening of the hospital later still, and the medical school last of all.

When Welch arrived in Baltimore in the fall of 1885 the only part of the university in actual being was the faculty of philosophy, already nine years old. He then took up various researches, some of them in collaboration with the nonmedical professors, and gave for four years informal but very fruitful instruction to a number of men who already had their M.D.'s, before the opening of the hospital to patients in May 1889; and thereafter confined his activities to the hospital until the inauguration of the medical school in the fall of 1893.

Owing to this sequence of events, the only affiliations that Welch could form on his first arrival were with the university proper and the scientists on its faculty; and this list toward science, rather than toward medicine narrowly conceived, was already an intrenched bias of work in the hospital on the very day that it opened its door to the sick. Another period of intrenchment followed, of the idea of a hospital alert to scientific issues and researches. And only when such a hospital so conducted had begun to make its mark and loom up as an institution that could not possibly be ignored or subordinated did the medical school itself begin to operate. The success of the Johns Hopkins University was a function of wise planning but also of beneficial delays.

The overlap between the different stages in the development of the full university structure was symbolized in the person of the physiologist H. Newell Martin, a professor in the faculty of philosophy with a claim to rank with Gilman, Billings, and Welch as one of the four principal founders of the medical tradition at Johns Hopkins. Welch's first assistant in pathology, the Baltimorean W. T. Councilman — a graduate of the University of Maryland Medical School and one of the few local men to receive positions of any distinction — had studied with Martin, and two of the first three preclinical professors in the medical faculty, when they came to be appointed, were his former students. Moreover, the two brilliant army surgeons, G. M. Sternberg (later Surgeon General) and Walter Reed, who by studying in Baltimore joined the traditions of the new university to those of the Army Med-

THE JOHNS HOPKINS HOSPITAL

ical Corps, received their first initiation into serious research under Newell Martin and only later came under the influence of Welch.

The link between Welch and Martin went beyond the setting of a tone and the recruiting by Martin of future students and colleagues for Welch and even beyond the part that Martin had played in passing upon Welch as a prospective appointee. The pathological laboratory at the hospital — a two-story building originally intended as a dead house — was not ready for occupancy when Welch first arrived, and he worked for a few weeks in Martin's laboratory. The episode was symbolic of the way in which the scientific researches of the two men meshed. Martin had devised in 1881 his method for perfusing the isolated mammalian heart and had made possible for the first time the study, from a physiological point of view, of the heart in isolation. Few contributions to physiology from an American laboratory have been of greater importance. Welch in particular was deeply impressed by Martin's work. In his own study of the alleged fatty degeneration of the heart as produced by heat, Welch cited, and repeated, the "positive proof" by Newell Martin in 1883 that the quickening of the pulse rate in artificially heated dogs and rabbits was due to the direct action of heated blood upon the heart. In men, in ideals, and even in research themes, the element of continuity between the laboratory of Newell Martin and that of Welch would be difficult to exaggerate.

The broader significance of this fact lay in the background from which Martin came — not German, but British. At the beginning of the 1870's T. H. Huxley had offered in London a famous laboratory course in general biology for teachers, with short talks followed by the dissection and sketching of various animals under the direction of a number of young assistants, of whom Newell Martin was one. Martin collaborated with Huxley in the preparation of a manual for such courses, which had a wide circulation throughout the English-speaking world. In this way he came to be recommended by Huxley as first professor of biology at Johns Hopkins. When to Martin's appointment is added the appointment of an Englishman as professor of mathematics and an American recommended by Clerk Maxwell as professor of physics, the conclusion is inescapable that though the Johns Hopkins University may have been in spirit the German university of America, the greatest proximate influence on the scientific side was British. Moreover, the major role played by Newell Martin in the prehistory of the hospital and the medical school meant that here also British influence was felt.

John Shaw Billings in particular, though aware of the strength of the German universities, strove consistently to redress the balance in favor of British models. After his first meeting with Welch in 1876 in Leipzig, he had written to Gilman apropos of the teaching of medicine there: "I have not yet seen any system of instruction which impresses me so favorably as that of Prof. [George] Rolleston at Oxford." His own choice of Welch as professor of pathology made it improbable that the Oxford system would prevail in Baltimore except by accident and indirection. But in one matter Billings was by common consent of Gilman and the trustees supreme and able to work his will for the long future: the ground plan and design of the great hospital to be built on spacious grounds in East Baltimore. The rambling structure which went up before Welch's eyes at the end of the 1880's — nasty red brick

THE JOHNS HOPKINS HOSPITAL

which nothing would ever mellow or soften, with a great central hall surmounted by a dome surmounted by a cupola surmounted by a spire — was the product of good will, inertia, and accommodation to the theories of disease of the pre-Kochian age from which Welch had just extricated himself at great cost.

Florence Nightingale had been appalled, with good reason, by the huddling together of throngs of ill-assorted patients in great barnlike structures and had laid down in the 1850's the dictum that hospitals ought to consist of a large number of "pavilions" or wards entirely separated from one another. "The object sought," she had written, "is that the atmosphere of no one pavilion or ward should diffuse itself to any other pavilion or ward, but should escape into the open air as speedily as possible, while its place is supplied by the purest obtainable air from outside." The military hospitals of the Civil War, the formative period in the life of Billings, were built on the pavilion plan of Florence Nightingale.

The same conception was now borne forward, after much patient investigation, into the building of the Johns Hopkins Hospital. The separate pavilions had a connecting corridor on the ground level, with one-story wards above. Though the corridor was continuous, the wards were not; and one could only get directly from ward to ward by walking through the open air on the floor formed by the ceiling of the corridor below. To get from the corridor to any of the wards, one had to take an outside staircase to the open-air walk above; and elevators were deliberately omitted so that stretchers would be carried up the outdoor stairs and no air be allowed to pass from the corridor to the ward. The pervasive note of the whole plan was a commitment to the transmission of disease by poisonous miasmas of the kind favored as carriers before the germ theory came in.

If the hospital plant was a monstrous anachronism, the implications of bacteriology for the architecture of hospitals had nowhere as yet been drawn forth; nor had the relative unimportance of the air transmission of germs been fully demonstrated. And the open-air walks made a pleasant place for sunning the patients. If the men and women who came to work in the wards and clinics were forward-looking, the fact that the hospital itself was backward-looking would make no real difference. As the building of the hospital progressed, the necessity of filling out the staff became urgent.

The choice of these people did not lie with Welch but with Billings; and to a hospital plan of British origin he now proposed to add a Scots chief surgeon, Sir William Macewen of Glasgow, the successor of Lord Lister. Macewen accepted the invitation on the condition that he be allowed to bring his own nurses with him and retain them entirely under his own control. The trustees were apprehensive in general about building a nest of young Nightingales, fearless and self-willed, and had no intention of putting into the hands of women the advantage of a divided sovereignty. The negotiations therefore fell to the ground.

Macewen was a great surgeon, but Welch had an alternative candidate of at least equal abilities and much broader range. Of the triumvirate who had built a shadow medical college of New York on German principles in the early eighties, Welch and Prudden had gone from one success to another. But the brilliant surgeon Halsted, with his bold slashing technique and open personality, had dropped away into tragedy and oblivion. In the fall of 1884, shortly after Welch left for his year in Europe, Carl Koller announced his discovery of cocaine as an agent for anesthetizing the eye. Halsted, with his assistants at the Roosevelt Hospital, at once took up the investigation of cocaine and made the discovery, laying the foundation for a theory of local anesthesia, that cocaine injected into the trunk of a sensory nerve produces insensitivity in the region to which the branches of the nerve spread out. The general use of local anesthetics began with this work.

The discovery came at too high a cost for Halsted himself. He and his assistants began to sniff cocaine up the nostrils and found that their minds became clearer and clearer, with no sense of fatigue and no desire or ability to sleep, but no sense of exhaustion on the morning after, the perfect antidote for the tireless activity of Halsted — until all of them had become addicts, progressively slowing down in everything they thought and did and grinding to a halt as effective human beings, a new kind of living dead. The evocation in literature of this first period of playing around with cocaine was Sherlock Holmes (first appearance in print 1887), who by edict of Conan Doyle escaped the consequences; in real life the genius who took to cocaine and went under was Halsted.

In 1885 he was induced to go for a year to Butler Hospital in Providence, the leading private institution in America for the care of mental disorders. This was the man, substantially written off by the medical profession, whom Welch invited in December 1886 to live with him in Baltimore and work in his laboratory. After one lapse, Halsted settled permanently in Baltimore at the end of 1887 — the only man among the early cocaine addicts to go on to a more brilliant career than before.

Most of him had died in the process, and he was now a new man: withdrawn, with a wary look, all the fire in him deliberately covered over by a sheet of ice, slow-moving beyond all endurance — so that a "Halsted" became a synonym for an operation drawn out to interminable length — tired, courteous, and infinitely patient. "Would you mind moving a little?" he said to one of his assistants after a long operation. "You've been standing on my foot for the last half hour." In outward things the old Halsted lived on only in his wardrobe: dozens of suits with irregular handsewn seams from London, shoes — cut from a place on the skin designated by himself — and shirts from Paris. Like some of the Russian aristocracy before 1914, he regularly sent his shirts to be laundered by Charvet in Paris and expressed surprise in later life on learning that there were thought to be good laundries in America. The new Halsted that dressed like the old had many foibles, much difficulty in making contact with other people — and great genius. Only Welch saw this from beginning to end and by an inspired exercise of faith and charity at the one critical moment knew how to salvage the greatest surgeon, taken all in all, America has ever seen. Welch procured Halsted's appointment as Associate Professor of Surgery in October 1889. The shadow medical college of New York was to be made visible in Baltimore. For the rest of his life Halsted's favorite subject of conversation was the merits of Welch.

The other major figure on the clinical side, the professor of medicine, was also a man whom Welch had known for some time, though not intimately — William Osler, who had gone from Montreal to Philadelphia and the University of Pennsylvania Medical School; "a well-knit but rather spare figure, of about the average height, a rather long moustache, the position of the ends of which seemed to vary with his mood; hair even then a little spare, a clear but rather sallow complexion, a broad forehead, good eyes and lively expression," a careful dresser with a taste for striking neckties.

If everyone has a characteristic situation in which he is most himself and least like anyone else and renews his image of himself by filling out the whole mold of his chosen personality, this situation for Osler was the tearing up of roots, a dread of security and an emotional compulsion toward rootlessness or — what came to much the same thing — toward the most diffuse possible kind of rooting. He had been successful and at least moderately happy in Philadelphia, but in 1888 his own recurring situation came up again with an invitation from Billings to become professor of medicine at Johns Hopkins. Osler accepted at once; his first communication to the provost of the University of Pennsylvania was a statement that he was leaving. Welch had felt from the outset that Osler was, as he wrote to his sister, "the best man to be found in the country." But Osler could not be, and was not, Welch's man in the same sense that Halsted was.

Osler had studied abroad but not for very long, and never formed really close ties with the scientific community in Germany. In so far as he represented directly any European traditions, they were those of the English hospital schools and the Scots universities as transplanted to Canada. The remaining member of the Big Four at the

Hopkins, Howard A. Kelly, initially associate professor of gynecology and obstetrics, was entirely American in training, experience, and outlook. He was a graduate of the University of Pennsylvania Medical School in the class of 1882 and had served as prosector to one of the great paleontologists of the nineteenth century, Joseph Leidy. On his own initiative Kelly built up a hospital in the outlying community of Kensington and began the brilliant operations that made his name — twinkling fingers "in and out of an abdomen almost before you knew it," abdomens flawlessly laid open in the moment required for an assistant to turn his back and thread a needle. From Kensington, Kelly felt the "Osler breezes" blowing from the university, and Osler for his part went to see Kelly operate and announced that he was backing a dark horse, a "Kensington colt," for the chair of obstetrics at Pennsylvania. He never stopped backing the Kensington colt; and Kelly always remained, in the ultimate things, Osler's man as Halsted was Welch's.

When Osler moved on to Baltimore, neither Billings nor Welch knew Kelly, and their only merit lay in taking Osler's advice to bring him on from Philadelphia. He was then thirty-one, an incomparable craftsman in a field where mere craftsmanship was no reproach but almost the highest praise, a magician with all of his magics deployed from the beginning, with no great capacities or need for growth. The only commonplace intellect among the Big Four, and the only conventionally devout man, with a consuming hatred of vice, drink, and graft, he always conducted a prayer-meeting for nurses, surgeons, and observers before operating. He was almost certainly the only member of the Big Four capable of addressing an assistant, without intending to be facetious, as "Brother Tom." He was also the only one to whom a nickname was never given by the students in general. Welch was "Popsy" behind his back; Halsted, "the Professor"; and Osler, "the Chief." But except to a very few, Kelly was Dr. Kelly. With patients he had difficulty in making them believe that he *was* a doctor, with his slight build and boyish face, sometimes but not always disguised by a drooping dark mustache. On one of the days when he had imprudently shaved it off, an old lady said to the intern, "You can't fool me, that boy's not Dr. Kelly."

President Gilman himself undertook to find the last of the men absolutely necessary for the functioning of a hospital, the superintendent, and chose the head of an insane asylum in Pontiac, Michigan, Henry M. Hurd. Then forty-six, and the oldest of the medical faculty, tall, thin, and solemn-looking but kindly, with side whiskers of an awkward cut, Hurd was a well-known figure in American psychiatry, the old psychiatry of the nineteenth century in which men of great intelligence worked diligently to no purpose at all for want of theoretical insight. But the best of the asylums supplied excellent training in hospital administration of a kind that was not afraid of innovations and endeavored at least to be rational and scientific; and Hurd at Johns Hopkins proved to be the ablest hospital superintendent of his time in America.

With the opening of the hospital to patients in May 1889 and the accompanying increase in staff, a critical period for Welch's influence at Johns Hopkins had begun. Up to this point the only men of at all comparable stature in Baltimore had been Halsted and Councilman, and one of these regarded Welch as a savior and the other was his second-in-command. Moreover, Welch was essentially a laboratory man who must now cease to live in the exclusively laboratory environment to which he had grown accustomed.

The history of the hospital from its opening in the spring of 1889 to the inauguration of the medical school in the fall of 1893 was notable for four things: the creation of a nurses' training school regarded for the first time in America as an integral and indispensable part of a hospital from the start; the beginning of a program of scientific publications in medicine; the institution of certain new departures in hospital administration and the care of patients; and the diffusion through the hospital of a commitment to research and laboratory work. The credit for the training school belonged to Gilman and Billings; and the founding of *The Johns Hopkins Hospital Bulletin* was the work of Hurd, who had before him the example of Gilman and the faculty of philosophy in launching a whole series of learned periodicals. The other two achievements may be divided among Gilman, Osler, and Welch.

The principle, always commented upon by students and visitors alike, of vesting almost unlimited power in the heads of departments and making them essentially independent of one another, may be credited in part to Gilman. But one of the two great contributions of William Osler to the history of the Johns Hopkins University lay in proposing the additional feature, unprecedented in the English-speaking world though familiar in Germany, of resident assistants to the departmental heads, with indefinite tenure and full authority in the absence of their chiefs. By this device, Osler remedied the radical defect in American hospitals of having no intermediate grade between many short-term interns and a few senior men on permanent tenure.

Good organization could foster whatever spirit happened to be moving in the hospital, but could not of itself supply ideals or final commitments. This definition of ends toward which the hospital community could be set in motion was the work in which Welch must take the lead or be increasingly overshadowed by the clinical staff.

Even before the opening of the hospital he had supplied a lodging place for Halsted and strengthened him in his native impulse toward becoming the most scientifically minded of all American surgeons. A fellow in pathology chosen by Welch, Franklin P. Mall, pointed out to Halsted in Welch's laboratory that the submucosa of the bowel wall was stronger than the mucosa and that intestinal stitches to hold should enter the former; and thus inspired the "Halsted suture." Halsted went on conferring with Mall for the rest of Mall's life. Welch therefore added to his initial service of saving Halsted as a human being, the creation of a research atmosphere which helped to give Halsted his distinctive attribute among great surgeons, of being more at home in the laboratory than in the surgery. Even in professional matters Welch exerted a decisive influence upon the chief surgeon of the Johns Hopkins Hospital.

Welch also made himself felt in Howard Kelly's department of gynecology and obstetrics. In 1892 a spare young man with black hair and the beak of an eagle, named Thomas S. Cullen, had come on from Canada with a view to working under Kelly. He began, however, by studying with Welch, and later, after a period in Europe, spent three more years in the pathological laboratory. When in the end he moved on to the operating theater he took with him the conviction that no one should qualify in gynecological surgery without first spending a year in gynecological pathology under Welch. To this Kelly agreed and so gave to Welch, and his successors, the opportunity of leaving an impress on every subsequent resident in gynecology. Even before the opening of the medical school, Welch had therefore begun to bring a second surgical department within his sphere of influence. In addition, when Kelly made over the field of obstetrics to another man in 1899, the new professor, J. Whitridge Williams, had begun his career by spending much time in Welch's laboratory and always retained an interest in pathology as the field of his first researches.

In one sense the clinical colleague whom Welch influenced the least as a professional man was William Osler — partly because Osler was already a convert to the things that Welch stood for. Yet one symbol of Osler's "science" in the eyes of his students was his insistence that in fevers they should always look under the microscope for the newly discovered malarial parasite. Osler had done research of his own on malaria before coming to Baltimore and would probably have given his students the same training in any circumstances. But in this context they and he could not fail to be impressed by the important investigations of malaria being pursued in Welch's laboratory and in particular Councilman's discovery in 1887 of malarial crescents.

Welch was a laboratory man capable of mastering a more than laboratory environment. The fact that he easily held his own with three great clinical men in their native milieu of a hospital not yet fitted into a medical school may well be the best possible index of his power in any situation to make his own ideals the core about which everything else compacted itself. He more than anyone else had made Johns Hopkins a new kind of hospital in American experience — the home not only of charity but of science.

VIII
A Very Happy Band

Though the Johns Hopkins Hospital was an excellent proving ground for Welch as a leader of men, and stood for great innovations in itself, it was not meant to stand alone. The whole intellectual structure was in danger without a medical school. But the funds intended for this purpose were invested in securities of the Baltimore and Ohio Railroad, which after a period of shrinking dividends made no payments at all from 1888 to 1891. Meanwhile other institutions saw their opportunity and both Pennsylvania and Harvard tried to lure Welch and Osler away. They refused, but could not be expected to wait for ever.

The solution had begun to work itself out as early as 1890. What the trustees of the university had not been able to do, their daughters did. In the process Johns Hopkins became involved in feminism. M. (for Martha) Carey Thomas, a brunette with a firm jaw and disenchanted look, was the member of a Quaker family in Baltimore, who tried in vain to be admitted as a regular graduate student in the university of which her physician father was a trustee. She took her doctorate instead at Zurich. From

1884 she was professor of English at Bryn Mawr College, but much in Baltimore with her friends Mary Gwinn, Mary Elizabeth Garrett, and Elizabeth King, whose fathers were or had been trustees also.

Miss Garrett was a soft, womanly-looking woman with a will of iron, the heiress of the president of the Baltimore and Ohio and his trusted adviser in business. She and Miss Thomas had collaborated in various enterprises, including the founding of a girls' school in Baltimore, and as early as 1889 Miss Thomas was proposing to take on the larger responsibility of finding money for the Johns Hopkins medical school. A year later she assumed a major role in the formation of a national Women's Fund Committee devoted to raising the necessary money, on the condition that women be admitted to the medical school on the same — *not* equal — terms with men. The list of subscribers rang with dynastic and almost institutional names like Adams, Bonaparte, Biddle, Drexel, and Widener, but also included Mrs. Louis Agassiz (the founder of Radcliffe), Mrs. S. Weir Mitchell, and Mrs. S. W. Gross (later Lady Osler); the First Lady Mrs. Benjamin Harrison; the celebrated women doctors Emily Blackwell and Mary Putnam Jacobi (the wife of Welch's friend at Bellevue); Alice Longfellow — "sweet Alice" — Julia Ward Howe, and Sarah Orne Jewett. The whole enterprise, with the judicious and almost cynical admixture of women of family with women of intellect, was a critical episode in the history of American feminism.

With almost $50,000 from Miss Garrett, the Women's Committee was able to offer to the trustees in the fall of 1890 the sum of $100,000 — if the admission of women were conceded. Miss Thomas always said that President

Gilman was utterly opposed to letting the women in "and used every unfair device — and he had many in his bag of tricks — to persuade the trustees to refuse this $100,000." He did not, however, choose to make his opposition public. The one leading figure at Johns Hopkins who took up a position of open hostility to the innovation was Welch. In later years he claimed that he had been troubled at the thought of saying things in the classroom that women would regard as indelicate. Hurd, Kelly, and Osler (no feminist) joined in advising the trustees to accept the initial gift of $100,000, but Welch refused to go along. The trustees followed the advice of the majority, and Welch soon admitted that he had been entirely mistaken.

Acceptance of the women's gift carried with it the proviso that the school should not be opened until the sum of $500,000 was obtained. Further efforts were therefore made by the Women's Committee, but more than $300,000 was still needed in December 1892. Miss Garrett then announced her willingness to make up the difference, and ended by having given from beginning to end a total of about $355,000. What the Baltimore and Ohio had put in peril, the Baltimore and Ohio saved.

Miss Garrett, however, had laid down conditions that caused Welch some embarrassment. Soon after coming to Baltimore he had drawn up for Gilman and the trustees a statement of the proper terms of admission to the projected medical school. These included the knowledge of chemistry and biology to be had by attending a good college, some acquaintance with Latin, mathematics, and physics, and an easy reading knowledge of French and German. Miss Garrett's conditions embodied the substance of Welch's own proposals as she understood them. "She naturally supposed," Welch wrote in 1922, "that this was exactly what we wanted." But he went on to say: "It is one thing to build an educational castle in the air at your library table, and another to face its actual appearance under the existing circumstances. We were alarmed, and wondered if any students would come or could meet the conditions."

Welch and his colleagues felt that Miss Garrett was attempting to bind them too closely, and perhaps for all time to come, to the then existing requirements in chemistry and biology in the college at Johns Hopkins; and he and the others did not relish the thought of a surrender by the faculty of their right to lay down their own requirements. Welch played a conciliatory role in the ultimate resolution of the difficulties. Though he and Gilman did not show the enthusiasm which would have been appropriate on having their own ideals held up before them as a standard, they did not propose a lower standard. Indeed, the net result of the controversy was the requirement that entering medical students should be graduates of a college of the first class rather than merely matriculants who had taken certain courses in science. Miss Garrett's standard had been raised, not lowered. But Gilman and Welch might never have had the courage of their own convictions without pressure from Miss Garrett and Miss Thomas.

The upshot was that the Johns Hopkins Medical School was the first in America to require a bachelor's degree and knowledge of French and German for admission. The unprecedented character of these requirements Osler summed up by saying to Welch, "Welch, we are lucky to get in as professors, for I am sure that neither you nor I could ever get in as students." The fact that the statement was false did not weaken its point.

Now that the necessary funds were available, the task of choosing the preclinical professors in anatomy, pharmacology, and physiology, fell primarily on Welch's shoulders. The Johns Hopkins University already had on its faculty one of the most distinguished physiologists of his time, Newell Martin, and the expectation had been that he would teach physiology in the medical school when it opened in the fall of 1893. But by the spring of that year he had sunk into hopeless alcoholism, and Osler undertook the awkward business of inducing him to resign rather than be dismissed; the saddest case he had ever known, Welch called it, and perhaps he thought of what Halsted might have been without himself. But Martin had left his mark on the medical traditions of Johns Hopkins, and two of the three preclinical professors chosen by Welch were former students of his — John J. Abel in pharmacology and William H. Howell in physiology. Abel, not quite thirty-six, handsome with a full beard and a Germanic look, after graduating from the University of Michigan had studied with Martin in Baltimore and then spent seven years under Ludwig, Schmiedeberg, Wagner, and many others in Germany. In breadth of training he was undoubtedly the best prepared of all the medical professors at Johns Hopkins. Howell, thirty-three years old in 1893, with a large spiked mustache, had taken his bachelor's and doctor's degrees at Johns Hopkins and risen to associate professor under Martin before accepting calls first to Michigan and then to Harvard.

Both at the time and in retrospect, Welch's greatest triumph lay in securing as professor of anatomy Franklin P.

Mall, the young man with whom Halsted had struck up a friendship in Welch's laboratory in the 1880's. Still only thirty-one in 1893, Mall was a small, spruce man, with a good smile and a sharp tongue; in physical appearance, a boy masquerading as a man with the help of a mustache. After graduating from the medical school at Michigan, he had done brilliant work in Leipzig under Carl Ludwig and the great embryologist Wilhelm His. Ludwig probably felt more respect and affection for Mall than any other student in the endless procession that wound through his laboratory over a period of fifty years. Under Ludwig, Mall carried through a masterly investigation of the structure and functioning of the intestine and built up a diagram of the supply of blood to the intestine, which led Ludwig to say of him that he had the true *Raumsinn,* the power to see structure in three dimensions, that distinguished the great anatomists from the competent. Mall said of himself that he would have liked to be an architect. In the course of his researches on the intestine he developed the important conception of "structural units" in an organ, the ultimate functioning units of which the organ is built up by repetition. He concluded that for the small intestine these were the villi — minute fingerlike projections from the intestinal wall, through which nutriment is absorbed.

With these superb investigations already behind him, Mall had worked from 1886 to 1889 as a fellow in pathology in Welch's laboratory. He then went to the new Clark University, only to participate in the historic dispersion by which the still newer University of Chicago "abducted" most of the brilliant faculty gathered together in Worcester. In Chicago, Mall met with instant recognition and helped to stimulate much grandiose talk of a medical school in Chicago better than Johns Hopkins and bigger and richer. How easily you talk of millions, Welch wrote to him gently! In the end Mall sent a telegram: SHALL CAST MY LOT WITH JOHNS HOPKINS. "Beside the magnificent opportunities at Baltimore," he wrote to Welch, "I consider you the greatest attraction. You make the opportunities."

With Mall, Abel, and Howell all of the initial high-level appointments to the Johns Hopkins Medical School had been made, and not one was a mistake. Gilman, Billings, Welch, and Osler among them had recruited a staff of which not one man was less than first rate. In retrospect they included the best pathologist, the best surgeon, the best clinician, the best gynecologist, the best anatomist, the best pharmacologist, the best hospital administrator, and the second or third best physiologist in America. From beginning to end, in donors, trustees, administrators, advisers, professors in the faculty of philosophy, and professors in the medical school, scarcely one undistinguished man or woman or person of limited vision had played an important role in the building of the university structure.

In the eyes of prospective appointees this sense of an appropriate context for their work, of a uniform environment with an equable climate of first-rateness, gave to the Johns Hopkins the prospect of durability in strength which it had to have to pull even with older institutions. Any impression of stumbling would have been fatal. The wise choices were cumulative, and drew one another after them, so that on the medical side the initial appointment of Welch was the pivot on which the whole success turned. By his own continued presence, despite opportunities to go elsewhere, Welch more than any other man gave to the medical faculty the corporate morale needed for holding firm under outside pressures.

The men of Johns Hopkins had been recruited for their independence of mind and spirit; and such men might have gone their separate ways in juxtaposition but not in unity, a community of the unclubbable with nothing in common but the interest of each in his own researches. The administrative setup, with its provision of near autonomy for heads of departments, pointed in this direction. But in fact they both formed clubs on a superficial level and at a deeper level participated in a common spirit over and above an interest in research.

The distinctive thing for which they stood and knew that they stood may be conveyed summarily by saying that when John Dewey came to enunciate his philosophy of education his ideals had already been acted upon in the Johns Hopkins Medical School. When early in the twentieth century all other medical schools in America were advised to make themselves over on the Hopkins pattern, it was no accident that the spokesman for this view turned to John Dewey for an elucidation of what the experiment in Baltimore amounted to. "Science," Abraham Flexner quoted Dewey as having written, "has been taught too much as an accumulation of ready-made material, with which students are to be made familiar, not enough as a method of thinking, an attitude of mind, after the pattern of which mental habits are to be transformed." Dewey, himself a Ph.D. made in Baltimore, was not referring to the Hopkins; nor had he inspired Welch and the other members of the medical faculty. They were influenced rather by the German laboratory tradition and the "inductive" teaching of biology by Huxley and Newell Martin.

The Hopkins temper in medicine involved a commitment to the process of learning by doing, as a means to the end of producing in students a generalized capacity to deal with problems scientifically; not particular problems defined — and resolved — in advance, but all problems, and real problems, with the unexpectedness about them that makes life different from school. As Mall put it, he did not want to produce "a shoemaker-physician who will drift into ruts and never get out of them." The majority of students were seeking a certain amount of information, preferably by drill, had little interest in "the solving of problems and the development of reason," and "mistook versatility for power." But a university must carry on "perpetual warfare against drilling trades into inferior students" and see that the medical profession was filled "with learned men, and not tradesmen." Though Mall was the most biting spokesman for this philosophy of education, Welch and most of the others were in perfect agreement with him. No charge infuriated Welch more than to be told that the Hopkins system was adapted only to the brilliant student who intended to be a scholar. He rejected the argument that there ought to be two kinds of medical instruction — "one designed for mediocre students to make practitioners, and the other for superior students to make investigators and teachers." On the contrary, "the practitioner is all the better if he has acquired by example and precept, something of the scientific spirit and attitude of mind, and the clinician, who becomes an investigator and teacher, should become interested in patients and know how to diagnose and treat their diseases."

The assumption was that habits of mind tended to generalize and diffuse themselves and break over from the laboratory into the clinic and the surgery and from one field of investigation into another. The generality, and almost the abstractness, the procedural rather than the substantive emphasis in this philosophy of medical education had many sources; but above all the interchangeability and flexibility of the personnel.

Welch had chosen as his title "professor of pathology" in place of the customary "pathological anatomy" (in America) and "pathological anatomy and general pathology" (in Germany). At the end of his life he wrote that he had done this "to stake out the claim that the chair really should cover, even if it did not actually cultivate, the whole broad field of the origin and nature of diseases." Thus he deliberately suppressed the emphasis on anatomy and by implication gave equal importance to physiology and bacteriology.

On the other hand, Mall, the favorite American student of the greatest teacher of physiology in Europe, figured on the Johns Hopkins faculty as professor of anatomy. When he began to teach gross anatomy in Baltimore he had not performed a dissection since his student days at Michigan and made rather rough weather of it for a while.

To complete the confusion, Osler before going to Philadelphia had been notable chiefly as a pathologist. His call to the clinical chair at the University of Pennsylvania had aroused much criticism as "the selection of a young man more known for his scientific papers than as a clinician." Halsted had always been a surgeon, but a surgeon of such breadth that he could easily have passed for an anatomist or a physiologist; and the pharmacologist Abel had mastered almost every conceivable branch of medicine.

With the possible exception, therefore, of Kelly, Hurd, and Howell, every member of the medical faculty could have performed the duties of one or more of his colleagues — and probably with great distinction. They naturally took for granted that new skills were easily acquired by the right sort of man. In 1897 Halsted ran into one of his assistants in the corridor — literally — and told Hugh Young to take charge of the department of genitourinary surgery. "I thanked him and said, 'This is a great surprise. I know nothing about genitourinary surgery.' Whereupon Dr. Halsted replied, 'Welch and I said you didn't know anything about it, but we believe you could learn.'" Young did, and became the greatest of all American urologists. The unspecificity of skills and powers was a living experience among the medical faculty.

The students for their part were expected to acquire the capacity of passing readily from one field of medical science or practice to another through experience in the actual confrontation of problems on their own, with the insight which this gave into the resolution of problematical situations in general. Both Osler and Mall, in many respects the polar opposites of the medical faculty, owed their distinctive place in the Hopkins tradition to this conviction.

Osler said of himself that he desired no other epitaph than to have "taught medical students in the wards." Under the system introduced by him and later imitated in every other American medical school of the first rank, medical students in their fourth year worked as surgical dressers and clinical clerks on the British model; with the difference that clear lines of authority, as in German hospitals, ran downward from the clinical chiefs through residents and assistants to the students themselves. To facilitate study in the wards under this scheme, Osler also introduced teaching laboratories into the hospital. Clinics, and at least nominal opportunities to visit hospitals, had long been known in American medical schools; but medical students as part of the functioning staff of a hospital, and the hospital itself as a college, were entirely new. "An old method," Osler wrote — and meant by this that it was old in the British Isles — "it is the only method by which medicine and surgery can be taught properly, as it is the identical manner in which the physician is himself taught when he gets into practice." This innovation of itself would have made the founding of the Johns Hopkins Hospital one of the great divides in the history of American medicine; and the whole meaning of it was to learn by doing.

In the department of anatomy, Mall conceived teaching to mean that he should put in the hands of every student a knife and part of a cadaver and then go away and let each man learn to swim by swimming. One of his settled convictions was that everybody teaches himself, or not at all, and has to be kept from leaning on crutches like detailed instruction from professors or the reading of Gray's *Anatomy,* which he forbade in his laboratories. He never gave a lecture — some said that this was because he himself was a miserable lecturer — or indulged in any other form of spoon-feeding. The poor and average students feared and hated him for this, but Gertrude Stein, the type of the student too brilliant to succeed in medical school, "delighted" in him. It was to her — but might have been to any one — that he said: ". . . nobody teaches anybody anything, at first every student's scalpel is dull and then later every student's scalpel is sharp, and nobody has taught anybody anything."

Though Mall's sarcastic tongue was resented, his real offense in the eyes of most students lay in his mode of teaching by not teaching. With this "inductive" method of instruction, which he thought of himself as having copied from Huxley, Mall combined a resolute failure to teach anatomy — even after his own fashion — in its medical bearings. "He had broken the control of the surgeons over the anatomical departments, so good for surgery and so bad for anatomy, and he would not go back to the old ways." His intention at Johns Hopkins was to leave as many doors as possible still open before the students for as long as possible. He argued that his function was not so much to supply them with facts as to cultivate in them the capacity for finding facts as needed. "To establish the habit of observing and reflecting, while at work with the scalpel and the microscope, is of far greater importance to the student than memorizing the subject matter for the sake of a quiz, an examination, or some subsequent clinical study." The characteristic Hopkins note of *general* preparation had been raised by Mall to the highest conceivable pitch; so much so that it grated on the ears of the clinician Osler, to whom it was not uncongenial.

Welch who lived on terms of equal friendship with Osler and Mall joined with them in dethroning the formal lecture and bringing to the center of the stage work in the pathological laboratory and the dissecting rooms. Short, heavy, and bald, with bright blue eyes, dark beard, and small hands and feet, he would turn up before the class in pathology — or not, in which case an assistant would

A VERY HAPPY BAND

wait for a moment and then take over — without having looked up his subject in advance and often without knowing what it was supposed to be. After finding this out, if necessary, he would begin by talking without notes for twenty or thirty minutes, with a brief description and perhaps a drawing on the blackboard of the organ or organs in health, but chiefly a discussion of the pathological state with frequent allusions of a more or less historical character to older researches on the subject. He would then have his *Diener* Schutz distribute sections for staining and mounting and would move among the students discussing with them what they saw under their microscopes.

Most of the laboratory instruction he left to his assistants, first Councilman and later Simon Flexner, supplemented by the fallible but confident wisdom of Schutz; and he himself seldom performed the autopsies at which attendance was obligatory for the students. Unlike Mall, Welch did not keep any particular watch over his assistants to be sure that they forced the students to do their own work and learn from their own mistakes. But he himself remained aloof from the students — though friendly enough when approached — made few suggestions for research exercises, offered few recommendations for supplementary reading, and conveyed the unmistakable impression that he must not be consulted about trifles or constantly badgered for advice. The men who could, would learn by fending in great part for themselves; and in the process they would acquire something better than facts, a first entry into the solving of genuine problems on their own. But where Mall by making articulate this philosophy of throwing students back upon themselves had earned their fear or hatred and made necessary constant supervision by himself to see that no one let the bars down, Welch achieved substantially the same result, with no murmur of criticism, by the mere setting of a tone which imposed itself by common consent even in his own increasing absence from the classroom and laboratory. Everyone knew that Welch would never guide a student by the hand, and the other instructors in pathology wished to do as Welch did and the students were content to be done by as by him.

Osler, Mall, and Welch had all participated after their fashion in a massive displacement of the center of gravity in the teaching of medicine in America, from memorizing to understanding, from reading and listening to seeing and doing. On this account the Johns Hopkins Medical School had made out for itself as early as 1900 some claim to be the best system of medical instruction in the world — distinctly superior in several respects to the German universities, though inferior as a source of creative researches. The German universities gave ideal training to advanced students of high quality, and to these only. Welch, Osler, and Mall had contrived to give to the ordinary medical student at Johns Hopkins better training than his counterpart in Germany, where the system of clinical clerks and surgical dressers was unknown, the didactic lecture continued to thrive, and the laboratory exercises of the undergraduate in medicine tended to be mechanical, listless, and routine. In the sphere of medical instruction for average students, the passing of the Age of European Supremacy did not wait for 1914 or 1939. This was the true significance of the first twenty-five years of Welch's time at the Hopkins.

Yet for him and the others as human beings the meaning of these years was to be at the point of forward thrust,

A VERY HAPPY BAND

with everything falling easy to hand and all the checks and obstacles of life in full flight before them. For a while it looked as if nothing they did could not succeed. "To have seen in so many ways," Osler said in 1913, "the fulfillment of our heart's desire is more than we could have expected, more indeed than we deserved." "To have lived through a revolution, to have seen a new birth of science, a new dispensation of health, reorganized medical schools, remodeled hospitals, a new outlook for humanity, is not given to every generation." For the founders the golden age at Johns Hopkins never turned to iron: Osler and the rest had in his words "both the vision from Pisgah and the crossing the Jordan." They made for themselves one of the great corporate happy times of the nineteenth century, and the words that recur as they look backward from old age are happy, happiness — "a very happy band" — "if work does not bring happiness there is something wrong," and the staff was then happy — "those early years so full of happiness, so full of hope."

The emblem of this happiness was the appearance of Osler at the hospital door every morning a few minutes before nine, in silk hat and frock coat and carrying a stick, with a greeting for Hurd. Then he would spring along the corridor toward the wards, humming a tune, with one arm through that of his assistant and the other punctuating joyous greetings for students and nurses or thrown around someone's shoulder, with a snowball of people closing in around him as he burst into the ward. At the bedside his whole teaching was to use all five of the senses: see the patient lying low in bed "like a log," smell the peculiar aromatic odor of tapeworms, listen for the succussion splash in pneumothorax, touch, feel, taste; and always put questions — bearing in mind that life is infinite in variety, and a man who says he took his first drink of the day before breakfast is a heavy drinker *unless* he lives south of the Mason and Dixon line and there many people nerve themselves for a sober day by having one stiff drink the first thing in the morning. With a joke or a teasing remark — of the kind that Howard Kelly did not like to have made at his expense and knew how to stop at once by reaching over and chucking Osler under the chin — Osler would distract the patients from their hoarded-up complaints and use their moment of laughter and almost grudging implication in his own happiness to extricate himself and move on to another bed. Patients, students, nurses, and even colleagues lived for a momentary brush of the Osler touch, and forgot to remember that he economized his time to the utmost and never let anyone hold on to him for long.

Osler's happiness was instantly communicable to everyone and even therapeutic. Elsewhere, in the operating rooms, there was an unspoken contentment that meant nothing to the inert forms of the patients but everything to the younger surgeons, satisfaction in standards of perfection never deviated from, at the two extremes of Halsted — the most slow-moving and circumspect of surgeons, though fully as drastic as need be and the originator of the massive amputation of the breast — and Howard Kelly, the most dazzling and rapid of surgeons, but invincibly conservative in cutting only what need be cut and reluctant to remove a single ovary.

Halsted would hang by the hour over the old wooden operating table which he had brought back with him from Germany — a relic of the army hospitals of the Franco-Prussian War, with a deep trough for thorough irrigation of wounds and a hole for drainage purposes — intent as no surgeon had ever been before on clamping or tying off every bleeding point without exception, and fanatical in his determination that no tissue be crushed and that every cell be treated as if the whole life of the organism were contained within it. When the young Harvey Cushing came from the Massachusetts General Hospital to Johns Hopkins, he took for granted that a patient would go into shock after a major operation, and this would have been true with almost any other surgeon anywhere else. But not with Halsted.

Many years later Halsted asked a friend if he understood what had made the Johns Hopkins Hospital, and gave his own answer: "Here we are not afraid to try things." With Halsted the trying of new things extended from his revolutionary emphasis on aid to healing as part of the operation itself, through constant researches in the laboratory — in the course of which he initiated Harvey Cushing into animal experimentation — to the physical accouterments of the surgeons and nurses. The white gown was already coming into use about the time of the opening of the Johns Hopkins Hospital, but Halsted added the skull-cap and required that his men change all their clothes before operating. Though he did not use masks, he was swept along more or less by accident into one further innovation. When he took Wade Hampton's daughter Caroline into the operating theater as head surgical nurse she found that her hands could not stand the strong solution of carbolic acid from which she had to lift the instruments. Halsted had some rubber gloves made up for her use; and from this beginning they imposed themselves on the surgeons as well, and spread to every hospital in the world.

He and Miss Hampton were married in 1890, with Welch as best man.

According to one account, the inspiration for the rubber gloves came from those used by Welch in making autopsies. But Halsted owed to Welch something more important, the spreading of an experimental temper through the hospital structure; and without this Halsted could not have been, in his own secretive way, a participant in the general sense of happiness in their work that bound the members of the Hopkins community together.

Howard Kelly, the surgeon that Halsted had been and the opposite pole to the surgeon that Halsted now was, also profited from the environment which Welch more than anyone else created; and he owed his finest moment, the kind of moral occasion in which he liked to figure, to the spirit which regarded even failures as instructive experiments from which something might be learned. In one week in 1895, four out of five abdominal operations in Kelly's department were fatal, and he and his assistants met to discuss what they should do. Cullen, with his long exposure to Welch, said at once, "Report everything." Kelly agreed, and the Johns Hopkins Hospital did what few hospitals had ever done before, published a frank account — in its own journal — of a disastrous lapse of its own, with an explanation of the probable cause. Kelly, the type of the moral man among the members of the medical faculty, could not have been altogether happy in the many places where this kind of gesture was impossible.

The contagion of the happiness of the senior men was always at work, but never more than in three Monday evening meetings every month: two sessions of the Medical Society and one session of the historical club. Welch and

Osler almost never missed a meeting of either, sometimes read the principal papers, always joined in the discussion, induced famous men to come in from the outside, and gave to both organizations an impetus which was not spent fifty years later. The initiative in founding the historical club had been taken by Osler, who never missed an opportunity in walking the wards to speak of the history of medicine and urge the reading of medical classics. But Billings had urged instruction in the subject from the beginning of his association with the university; Howard Kelly became in time the biographer of Walter Reed and editor of the standard biographical dictionary of American physicians; and Welch served with great enthusiasm and success as first president of the society. The recollection that remained with the younger men for the rest of their lives was the fact that the two biggest men on the faculty, Welch and Osler, always found time to come in good weather and bad.

For *young* men — ranging in 1893 from Mall at thirty-one to Welch at forty-three and Osler at forty-four — this atmosphere of happiness that seemed for a long time to know no boundaries or diminution, but only spreading and increase, must almost have seemed the universal meaning of entering upon maturity, and not in any way local or private. One reason why the men of Johns Hopkins were happy above most men of their time lay concealed in the observation of the Boston surgeon Reginald Fitz, who came down to see and said that he had found a monastery in Baltimore. In a happy monastery men have an undistracted devotion to their calling, have fellowship and work together under discipline, but conduct in freedom their own transactions with the spirit that is in and above them, and know that to perfect themselves in the way to which they aspire as individuals will cause their ends to melt into the ends of the universe. The men of Johns Hopkins had this same sense that if they only did well what they would wish to do as individuals they would contribute to the happiness of everyone else.

Like religious men also, who believe in their own vision, the men and women of Johns Hopkins had an overflowing charity and wish to go among others and implicate them in a common well-being and condition of health and salvation. It was no accident that Welch took the lead in securing for the people of Baltimore a filtration plant for the city water supply and the delivery of Pasteurized milk in individual bottles; no accident that medical social service in America began in this context with the sending by Osler in 1898–1899 of two women medical students into the neighborhood around the hospital to give instruction in the home care of tuberculosis; no accident that another student who went out from the hospital to take her turn in delivering the babies of the poor, Gertrude Stein, first let the Negro speak in literature with the accents of life.

Unlike many religious bodies, the men of Johns Hopkins had the example of Welch, Osler, and Halsted (but not Kelly) to show that clothes and food and drink did not have to be put down but could be integrated into their professional lives; that fullness of being was no crime against their calling. Eating and drinking were simply pretexts for letting the life of the hospital go on out of hours. When Councilman was caught in an error, he would say, "B-b-boys, l-l-l-let's go over to the ch-ch-church," and everybody would run across to Hanselmann's Bar — "the church" — at the corner of Wolfe and Monument streets, and the shop talk would go on over the beer. Here Hanselmann had once run his hand over Halsted's head and cried out, "You have not approximately lost your hair," and Halsted had turned red and angry.

Better than "going to church" was an invitation from the three lavish hosts of the Big Four — Osler, who could make "beer, backy, oysters" at 1 West Franklin Street the occasion of a lifetime; Halsted, who chose a terrapin from the private stock in his cellar and served incomparable dinners of state, but did not know how to dispel the chill that hung over him and his aristocratic wife on social occasions; and above all Welch with the orderly gradation of his dinners at the Maryland or University Club, from a good meal but modest for minor visitors to terrapin and Madeira for luminaries of the first rank. The bachelor Welch, who always lived in a few rented rooms and entertained in the public atmosphere of a club, was in his element as host or master of ceremonies and transacted much of the business of the hospital and the medical school over dinner. Perhaps a man who had no private life except to be alone had for his own sake to make a success of entertaining and domesticating public occasions to his personal needs, as the ash from his cigar fell thicker and thicker on his clothes and the talk flowed on.

He, like Osler, shone also at ceremonial dinners. "Ten yurs at Johns Hopkins. Ten yurs at Johns Hopkins," the non-drinking member of the staff who got drunk for the tenth anniversary of the hospital ejaculated in response to a call for remarks and dropped back into his seat with a thud, and everyone began to imagine how the embarrassed silence would drag out to eternity. But Welch was on his feet at once to say, "A great thought, adequately expressed!" — and the tension broke in a roar of applause.

In his native milieu of the social occasion that needs to be warmed up and made easy, Welch never lost this art of breaking tensions and preserving in the Hopkins men their sense of fellow-feeling and common purpose.

What he had in mind above everything else as defining this purpose was the university connection making itself felt through the hospital and the medical school, and science and experimentation getting the better of empiricism and routine. In 1905 the least likely of all visitors came to see the hospital, and unknowingly passed his verdict on the whole effort that Welch had been making to keep this purpose alive. "Why should the great Hospital, with its endless chambers of woe . . . have turned . . . to fine poetry, to a mere shining vision of . . . the high beauty of applied science?" asked Henry James, and found his own answer. "It partook for me . . . of the University glamour," and made itself felt as an agent of "the higher tone" emanating from the "bland presence" of the university.

Henry James did not mention Welch by name, may never have known of his existence, and knew nothing about hospitals. But he had the intuitive sympathy to know at once when something ugly had been made not ugly and the care of misery and sickness transformed into a work of art; and then wrote the most eloquent and perceptive appreciation of Welch's life work that has ever appeared.

IX
The Laboratory Regimen in Baltimore

At Johns Hopkins and elsewhere in America the name of Welch was synonymous with the scientific ideal in medicine, almost from the moment of his arrival in Baltimore in 1885 till his death fifty years later. But a grave irony here lay concealed. For Welch had performed the last of his experimental researches before the opening of the Johns Hopkins Medical School in 1893; and by about 1900 had substantially abandoned even the low level of creativity in science which consists of synthesizing the literature of other people's researches. The verdict passed upon him in 1903 by his fellow workers as being the most distinguished American pathologist was even then profoundly retrospective. In his chosen field the future had slipped from his grasp a decade before. He had had about seven years of genuine research and conducted about half a dozen leading investigations, none of the first importance and all but one derivative.

The first of Welch's researches after settling in Baltimore touched upon one of the major themes in nineteenth-century pathology, Bright's disease of the kidney. In the production of urine a central role is played by the Malpighian bodies, each comprised of a tuft of capillaries, the glomerulus, enclosed within a capsule. Welch undertook, by administering poison to white rats and rabbits, to induce a diseased state of the Malpighian bodies, and succeeded in bringing about suppression of the urine. On autopsy the Malpighian bodies showed distinct changes from their normal condition. Welch attempted to set up a distinction between the pathological deposit of cells and granular material between the glomerulus or tuft of capillaries and the capsule enclosing it, on the one hand, and on the other hand similar deposits entirely inside the capillaries. For the latter type he proposed the name which caught on, of "intracapillary glomerulitis."

After this first trial flight, Welch took up in succession three researches which bore directly on the nexus of issues and egos that constituted the relationship of Virchow, Cohnheim, and von Recklinghausen. One of the really magisterial achievements of Virchow had been to create almost singlehanded the concept of thrombosis, the obstructing of the blood or lymph stream by plugs — thrombi — of various kinds. His greatest students, Cohnheim and von Recklinghausen, had had of necessity as part of defining their own personalities as investigators to take up positions on thrombosis. Cohnheim characteristically affirmed his maturity and independence of the master by arguing that Virchow had greatly underestimated the role played in thrombosis by changes in the walls of the blood vessels. Characteristically also, von Recklinghausen exercised his freedom from tutelage to reaffirm the traditional Virchowian view and to depreciate the importance of changes in the vessel walls. Welch, in setting forth the results of his work in the experimental production of thrombi in dogs, expressly took the side of von Recklinghausen against Cohnheim. The principal object of his research was not to pass upon this issue, but upon the claim made by two German investigators that the so-called "white" thrombi contain as essential constituents blood platelets only, and not fibrin or leucocytes (white corpuscles). Welch showed that all three constituents go to make up the white thrombus.

In 1877 when Welch was still a student at Breslau he had written to his father of Cohnheim's work with hemorrhagic infarction — a special form of thrombosis or embolism in which by obstruction of the flow of blood a region of local cell death occurs, accompanied by hemorrhage. Cohnheim attributed this condition, given the presence of an arterial thrombus or plug, to the reflux of blood from the veins toward the region of infarction, with hemorrhage resulting from the passage of blood corpuscles through the vessel walls into the surrounding tissues. Here as always he invoked an alteration in the vessel wall itself. But various publications from von Recklinghausen's laboratory undertook to show that the blood came not from the veins by reflux but from the collateral vessels, and that blood dammed up in the capillaries would cause hemorrhage by its increased pressure without any change in the walls. With the assistance of Franklin P. Mall, Welch now entered this controversy. Their conclusions directly contradicted Cohnheim and in all essential points confirmed the position of von Recklinghausen's associates.

Still a third investigation in which Welch confronted the authority of his old instructors was the study of heat as the causative agent in fatty degeneration of the heart. Von Recklinghausen and the celebrated clinician Bernard

Naunyn had challenged the conventional view that degeneration must follow excessive heat. Welch therefore subjected rabbits to temperatures ranging from 105 to 108 degrees Fahrenheit, and found that von Recklinghausen and Naunyn were wrong; but also that their antagonists in Europe were mistaken in supposing that fatty degeneration set in immediately after the application of heat. Welch found that a distinct interval was required.

All of Welch's remaining researches dealt with bacteriology. John Shaw Billings long before had called for the study of veterinary problems at Johns Hopkins, and Welch in investigations first published in 1889 and restated in 1894 addressed himself to the nature of hog cholera. He argued that "buttons" of the intestine characterize hog cholera as a famous intestinal lesion in man characterizes typhoid; and he showed that these buttons were produced by a particular bacillus. In fact hog cholera is caused by a virus, and the buttons are a secondary manifestation, not invariable, of a secondary invasion by bacteria.

In the bacteriology of human disease, Welch in publications begun in 1890 and completed in 1892 stated his conviction that the *pneumococcus* was the causative agent of lobar pneumonia; and together with his assistant Alexander C. Abbott demonstrated that Prudden was mistaken in saying that true diphtheria could be found in the absence of the Klebs-Loeffler bacillus. Work of this character, though valuable in shaping American opinion and putting down the suspicion that diphtheria in the New World might be a different disease from diphtheria in Europe, made no claim to originality.

Two concluding researches in bacteriology had greater freshness. In October 1891 a mulatto died in Osler's ward.

Welch, in the autopsy, found over large regions of the upper part of the body a distinct crackling sound under the touch. When he exposed the veins and arteries he could tell even before opening them that they contained large numbers of gas bubbles. On cutting the vessels he secured a gas burning "with a pale bluish, almost colorless flame, a slight explosive sound being heard at the moment of ignition." By further researches Welch and his assistant G. H. F. Nuttall discovered the bacillus responsible for producing the gas — called after him *Bacillus welchii*. His admirers liked to think of him as the founder of a new field of investigation, pneumopathology, and he undoubtedly added a new chapter to the history of emphysema — the swelling produced by gas in body tissues — and perhaps supplied a clue to the many historical accounts of "spontaneous combustion" in men.

Another research proved to have more important immediate consequences: the discrimination by Welch of *Staphylococcus epidermidis albus,* and the proof that it was present in the deeper layers of the skin and inaccessible on this account to surface disinfectants. The demonstration of this fact in 1891 led Halsted to make his important innovation of using subcutaneous stitches and merely drawing together the surface boundaries of the incision. In this way Halsted avoided the stitch abscesses then prevalent even in antiseptic surgery of the most painstaking kind. For the same reason, the presence of *epidermidis albus* as an inhabitant of the body already in residence, Halsted made famous the practice of allowing the empty spaces arising out of surgery to fill with blood clots. He thus avoided the introduction of various foreign materials, soluble and otherwise, but all of them adapted to becoming either foci or paths of suppuration. The absence of stitch abscesses and in general the avoidance of suppuration became an integral part of the Halsted technique in surgery. As Welch had saved Halsted from moral degradation and professional ruin, so Halsted gave to the researches of Welch their most practical application.

Bacteriology may well have been the field of biology with the lowest average prospect of attaining fresh insights as distinguished from particular new facts supporting the germ theory of disease. An estimate of the spontaneity and freshness of Welch's research must therefore rest on his investigations in the tradition of Virchow, Cohnheim, and von Recklinghausen, rather than of Koch. The trinity of researches into white thrombi, hemorrhagic infarction, and fatty degeneration of the heart all display a certain independence and a willingness to contradict at least one of his masters — sometimes Cohnheim, sometimes von Recklinghausen, but never as it happened both. But that he should go on walking the treadmill of issues defined by other men and restricting the exercise of his freedom to a choice among *their* alternatives was a sure sign that though he might be the conductor through whom the creative spark passed from Ludwig, Cohnheim, and von Recklinghausen to other Americans, he was not himself to be a true generator of fresh currents. Whether he would even be the conductor of the creative tradition would turn on the regimen of his laboratory.

As Welch knew from his time in Europe, the possession of a research laboratory was the possession of power, but a special kind of power of which the legitimate end could not be had by coercion. The laboratory director wishing to have creative students must provide and sustain, for their sake and his, a permissive environment. Welch in his own laboratory in Baltimore introduced a new magnitude of permissiveness, verging on the chaotic. Contrary to the usual practice in Germany, he set no common theme for his associates; and he continued, also in the face of the best German traditions, to serve as director after he had consciously withdrawn from research. With this withdrawal he combined the wise policy in the circumstances of permitting the workers in his laboratory to go their own way, unless they asked for advice.

Welch seldom formulated problems for his students. A joint investigation by him and his favorite pupil and colleague Simon Flexner — a small, almost elfin-looking man from Louisville, who had first come to Baltimore in 1890 as a graduate student in pathology — was a special case. The discoverer of the diphtheria bacillus, Friedrich Loeffler, had been unable to find in experimental animals a characteristic lesion of diphtheria in man; and in a research for which Flexner performed the experiments, he and Welch succeeded in demonstrating the existence of this lesion in lower animals as well. Their findings confirmed the view that diphtheria was essentially local in origin (within the body).

Welch's suggestions for research to be conducted by students on their own were few and generally abortive. In line with his own interests he suggested to Eugene L. Opie a study of the relationship of blood platelets to thrombus formation; but Opie had no success in the artificial production of thrombi outside the body and soon turned to other and more congenial problems. After a visit by Sir Almroth Wright, Welch suggested that George H. Whipple work on the "opsonins" discovered by Wright —

"buttering" agents in the blood serum which render bacteria susceptible to attack by white corpuscles. Whipple simply declined the invitation and continued his investigation of injuries caused by chloroform to the liver.

The two important suggestions for research made by Welch, and acted upon, fell outside the life of his own laboratory. In 1905 he urged Simon Flexner to begin work on the syphilis spirochete, and this impulse as transmitted by Flexner to an associate led to the proof by Hideyo Noguchi of the relationship of the spirochete to neurosyphilis, and in more general terms the building by Noguchi of a reputation as the leading American syphilologist. He had never studied with Welch.

After the triumphant conclusion of the labors of the Yellow Fever Commission, the causative organism of the fever, as distinguished from the insect carrier, still remained to be found. On this subject Walter Reed consulted his old instructor in Baltimore, and Welch called his attention to the proof by Friedrich Loeffler and Paul Frosch in 1898 that the foot and mouth disease of cattle is caused by a filtrable virus. Reed and his associate James Carroll (another former student at Johns Hopkins) followed up this clue and demonstrated in 1901 that a filtrable virus was also responsible for yellow fever — the first proof that a specific human disease was caused by a virus.

In general the men in Welch's laboratory uncovered their own problems in the flow of pathological materials from the hospital. "Dr. Welch did not seem to think that personal guidance of those engaged in research was desirable." On these terms the men sought him out when they had "something worth bringing," but only then. They soon learned that he would like to hear of fresh observations made by themselves; but that these would be subjected to a searching criticism and awkward questions thrown out to stick in their minds. Yet he "never dampened enthusiasm."

The result was a large number of valuable researches with no unifying theme and no great cumulative effect. The more important of these included: the discovery by W. T. Councilman in 1887 of the crescent phase of the malarial parasite; the discovery by Arthur G. Blachstein in 1890 of the chronic carrier of typhoid bacilli in the biliary passages and of the relationship between typhoid infection of the gall bladder and the formation of gallstones; a contribution by Councilman and H. A. LaFleur in 1891 to an understanding of the role of pathogenic amoebae in producing amoebic dysentery; the investigation by Walter Reed in 1895 of the lymphoid nodules of the liver in typhoid fever; the demonstration by T. S. Cullen in 1896 that adenomyoma of the uterus (a tumor developing as a muscular thickening of the inner wall of the womb) had its origin, in spite of the contrary opinion of von Recklinghausen, in the mucous membrane lining the uterus; the discovery by T. C. Gilchrist in 1896 of the skin lesions caused by the Blastomyces fungi; the first demonstration by W. G. MacCallum in 1897 of the sexual conjugation of the malarial organism, that is, the entrance of a flagellum or whip into the crescent of Councilman; the proof by Eugene L. Opie in 1901, by pathological microscopic studies, of a connection between the islands of Langerhans and diabetes in man; and the demonstration by MacCallum and Carl Voegtlin in 1908–1909 that removal of the parathyroid glands leads to a calcium deficiency and that the accompanying postoperative spasms may be controlled by the administration of calcium — the first insight into the function of the parathyroids.

Disjointed and lacking in direction as these investigations were, they nevertheless constituted a remarkable record for which much of the credit went to Welch and the "atmosphere" which he created. This almost obscurantist formula of "atmosphere" implied that Welch by the looseness of his control, combined with the attraction of his personality, had hit upon a new regimen of the laboratory from which creative minds could emerge intact. Welch's career is evidence that nearly absolute power need not corrupt, in the sense of working injury to others and depriving them of freedom. In part, the freedom in Welch's laboratory sprang from the fact that he soon branched out into many other undertakings, including the deanship of the medical school. Nobody can be an effective tyrant if he has too much authority in too many spheres. But though this dispersion of energies confirmed Welch in his natural inclination to let students go their own way in peace, it gave to him personally a sense of the divided and distracted will and a feeling almost of frustration.

In one way only he might have remained within the research enterprise, after his withdrawal from research itself: by the depth of his insight into biological problems on their philosophical side. But the only "idea" of theoretical import in his writings is evolution. His own favorite among the whole body of his publications was the address "Adaptation in Pathological Processes," with its central thesis that if the capacity of the organism to adapt itself to pathological conditions were perfect this could only be at the expense of the normal functions in health and would represent a drag on evolutionary progress. Not the higher, but the lower animals had the power to regenerate lost parts. Nothing truly comparable to this paper can be found elsewhere in Welch's writings. He was not fitted to be a philosopher of the biological sciences.

One poor substitute remained to give him a sense of active participation from within the research community, summarizing the researches of others. The last of his substantial contributions of this character was a lecture delivered in London in 1902, "On Recent Studies of Immunity." This able summary of the literature in a field which had just begun to come in when he abandoned research might well have seemed to Welch the ultimate degradation — a restatement of the findings of others, without the slightest admixture of his own work. But he was now too deeply involved in other things, and the habit of research had slipped away from him forever.

George Eliot — whose last books were published in Welch's early manhood and read by him — had portrayed as a symbol of moral disintegration in *Middlemarch* a student of the clinician Louis of Paris who turned aside from research to make money. Welch in his own person represented an enormous amplification of the moral dilemmas of a medical research man — many different ways of seceding from research, and all disinterested, but if treason to one's calling is either treason or not, treasonable.

Welch learned to live with his own response to this new human situation, a new predicament in the history of the inner life which he was almost the first American ever to experience. The miracle of the forty years which remained to him after his retreat from research was to go on projecting, with no trace of the fraudulent or hypocritical and no loss of fire or conviction, the ideal of research in medicine. The flame had not died of itself, or been blown out by others. Both in his own laboratory and elsewhere he found no estrangement from the men who were now doing what he too had done, but only for a short time in the receding past. He would speak his own verdict on himself only once in public, and when the time came no one would listen.

X
The Birth of an Influential

THE BIRTH OF THE TEXTBOOK in Hellenistic Alexandria was the first systematic recognition that the advance of science requires the forming of a consensus of expert opinion, intended not to repress innovation but to give to it point and zest and a prospect of general acceptance. Thereafter the pursuit of this consensus never ceased. The whole development bore with it one great political lesson: the necessity for the self-government of the scientific community and the emergence from within, by the unintimidated consent of the scientists themselves, of a body of Influentials who had the consensus in their keeping.

William Henry Welch had come by 1900 to fill the role of the leading Influential of American science in succession to Benjamin Franklin and the elder Benjamin Silliman of Yale — by far the greatest Influential that the biological sciences had yet known in America. Welch was president of the Association of American Physicians in 1901, president of the Board of Scientific Directors of the Rockefeller Institute from 1901 to 1933, president of the American Association for the Advancement of Science in 1906, chairman of the Executive Committee of the Carnegie Institution of Washington from 1909 to 1916, president of the American Medical Association in 1910–1911, president of the National Academy of Sciences from 1913 to 1916, and chairman of the Advisory Council of the Milbank Memorial Fund from 1922 to 1932. The list is not exhaustive but representative.

Certain of the responsibilities that Welch had entered upon as an Influential of the first magnitude have remained constant through the whole history of the consensus: the bestowal of the imprimatur of science upon some but not all observations and theories; the redistribution of emphases, as one field or mode of attack plays out and another is taken up; and the admission of newcomers to the scientific community, with a prima facie claim to be heard with respect, and thereafter a grading upward of successively smaller groups until only the Influentials of the next generation are left. The withdrawal of confidence from senior men, and less often their banishment, must also go forward, though always impeded if never checked for long by the fellow-feeling of the Influentials for men of their own age and rank.

The life of science as Welch had known it embodied in the laboratory regimen the type of the milieu where the best use of power was its own disuse; but in the forming of the consensus, the blade of power had to fall and cut and lop off without ceasing. Only the ruthless pruning of reputations could leave breathing room for the survivors. Choice there must be. But though the Influential could not avoid exercising power he might choose according to his temperament either to emphasize the unsoundness of bad work and poor men, or else to endorse these judgments in silence and press the claims of good work and good men. Welch chose the latter.

As director of the most famous teaching laboratory for pathology in America, he had the opportunity to examine at firsthand dozens of young investigators; and then by a nod of his head to place them in important positions throughout the country. For the first thirty years of his time in Baltimore few major appointments in pathology were made without consulting Welch. Of his own colleagues and students whom he launched on their careers — Welch rabbits — the best known included W. T. Councilman, chosen by Harvard to fill a post initially offered to Welch himself; Simon Flexner of the University of Pennsylvania and the Rockefeller Institute; Alexander C. Abbott of Pennsylvania; the Nobel prize winner George H. Whipple of California and Rochester; Milton C. Winternitz of Yale; Ernest Goodpasture of Washington University; Rufus Cole, Christian Herter, Eugene L. Opie, and Peyton Rous, all of the Rockefeller Institute; with others like Mall, Gilchrist, Whitridge Williams, Cullen, and MacCallum (who went for a time to the College of Physicians and Surgeons in New York, now truly a part of Columbia University), whom he kept at Johns Hopkins itself or brought back. In England his student G. H. F. Nuttall came by a roundabout process to be a professor in Cambridge University.

Welch as the greatest Influential of his time in America passed not only upon his own students and associates but upon others. Men as diverse as T. Mitchell Prudden, Alexis Carrel, and Hans Zinsser rose in public standing and self-respect by Welch's decree. The list of similar gestures of recognition by Welch, with their power to transform men's lives almost by a flick of his wrist, might be multiplied indefinitely. Two instances have the added interest of displaying the role which he had come to fill in public life during Theodore Roosevelt's administration.

As the time for building the Panama Canal approached, the commission in charge included several engineers but no physician, not even the great army sanitarian William C. Gorgas, whom Welch had had in his New York quiz a generation earlier. The engineers made light of the necessity for mosquito control of the kind through which Gorgas had driven yellow fever from Havana. Welch therefore wrote to President Roosevelt in 1904 to emphasize the importance of sanitary measures. Roosevelt at once transmitted the letter to the head of the commission with instructions to consult Welch.

Encouraged by this, Welch led a delegation to the White House and seized the opportunity to argue that Gorgas ought not only to be in charge of all sanitary measures but also a full-fledged member of the commission itself. Roosevelt was unable to comply because Congress had laid too many restrictions upon the engineering qualifications of the commissioners. For the time being, Welch had to be content with Gorgas's appointment as chief sanitary adviser. Welch's warning that without the prestige of a commissioner Gorgas would be hamstrung was amply fulfilled. After a visit to the Isthmus in 1907 the President appointed Gorgas to the commission. Welch then wrote to Roosevelt to say "virtually 'I told you so.'"

Another Roosevelt enterprise was almost as significant as the building of the Panama Canal: the appointment in 1906 of a Country Life Commission, to study the problems of rural living in America. A medical zoologist of the United States Public Health and Marine Hospital Service, who had been lecturing at Johns Hopkins since 1897, Dr. Charles W. Stiles, wanted to be on the commission in order to "do something for the 'poor whites' of the South." Like Gorgas he failed in his first attempt to be appointed; but a vacancy appeared almost at once, and Stiles invoked the aid of Welch. This time Stiles was chosen, and he moved toward the historic rendezvous when he sat up all night pouring forth to Wallace Buttrick the circular miseries of the poor white, kept by hookworm disease poor, lean, and languid, and by poverty and languor kept diseased; and found on the morning after that he had tapped the wealth of the Rockefellers for applying the remedy of purges, shoes, and privies.

It was part of Welch's retreat from research that he found judgments on men more congenial than judgments on scientific controversies. He did occasionally, as with a clinical report of his old friend Abraham Jacobi in 1895, reject out-of-hand findings which he thought unfit to be absorbed into the consensus. Like the whole scientific community, he also withheld from certain famous theories the full acceptance which their authors sought: of Paul Ehrlich's "side-chain" theory of immunity, he never said more than that it was a fruitful working hypothesis; and he went no further in discussing Elie Metchnikoff's "phagocytism" (the exclusive role of the white corpuscle in combating disease organisms) than to say that a case had been made out with great skill for the playing of an *important* role by the phagocytes. Here Welch performed the ironic task of an Influential like himself, of denying full entry into the scientific consensus of the ideas of men greater than himself in research and inspiration.

Welch's impulse as an Influential was in fact to rise

above the details of the consensus and discuss in broad terms how admission to it might be won. He seldom dealt in right attitudes and good prepossessions, but rather in suggestions for kinds of research — new areas of investigation, or old areas now unduly neglected. By suggestions of this character, Welch took part in the process by which the Influentials deploy as many kinds of troops as possible with a minimum of raggedness in the line of advance; tightening up — in terms of publishability and public recognition — the standard of significant work in a field which has been overcultivated; and making comparatively easy the attraction of attention by work in a field which has been neglected.

Thus, within the bounds of his own experience, Welch spoke in 1916 of the commanding importance of pathological anatomy, despite the relative neglect into which it had fallen with the rise of bacteriology, and held out to the bacteriologist with sound anatomical training the prospect of surpassing his rivals. In a field outside his own, he repeatedly called attention to the new development of tropical medicine, and induced the Surgeon General of the navy to send a man for training under Sir Patrick Manson in London. The man chosen went on to found a vigorous tradition of tropical medicine in the Naval Medical School.

As part of the same impulse to get men working in fresh or neglected fields, Welch often urged new medical schools to seize upon problems for which they had local advantages. Tulane, he said in 1914, should develop tropical medicine; Peking, in 1921, should make sure not to do merely the same kind of work on the same themes as Baltimore and Boston. By responsiveness to local conditions, the world-wide community of scientific medicine could be made self-correcting in its emphases and enthusiasms.

Much of the work of an Influential consisted in this way of a calculated shifting of his own weight. How seriously Welch took this responsibility may be seen with special clarity when he tried to redress the balance against himself. Thus he, who had come to be the symbol of laboratory instruction in medicine, pointed out as early as 1894 that laboratory teaching could be overemphasized. Without didactic lectures and textbooks, there would be a loss of perspective and a failure "to comprehend the general bearing of observed facts." At a time when the reforms associated with Johns Hopkins had nowhere been fully imitated, Welch had begun to warn against possible disadvantages of the Hopkins ideal if pressed too far. One chief task of the Influential, as he recognized, was to guard against his own successes. With Welch as with others, the character of a good Influential in science resembled that of a trimmer in politics.

In this way Welch performed the conventional tasks of the Influential. But in the increasingly elaborated scientific community of his time he could not have raised himself above the level of his rivals unless he had found new kinds of work to do and come to represent a new conception of the Influential's role. He struck the answering vibration to certain elements of novelty in the later nineteenth and early twentieth centuries: the recognition by many intellectuals that everywhere in the Western world the masses of men would have to be given social amenities as well as political rights; the growing awareness of the whole people as a force to be reckoned with; and the effort of the Gilded Age to transform itself into an Age of Philanthropy.

Welch in confronting "the social problem" as the leading spokesman for the medical profession in America had first to define and if necessary delimit the claim of the public health movement to be an agency of reform. Here he encountered the central equivocation of the reform impulse: whether the new beginning from which everything else would follow must come from a change of heart or a change of scene. On one side stood the whole body of religious opinion; on the other, the secular philosophy for which the nineteenth-century socialist Robert Owen had spoken long before in saying, "Man's character is made for, not by, him." The locus of intersection of the two philosophies was the Charity Organization movement, represented in Baltimore by a society founded in President Gilman's office, with active assistance from Hurd as superintendent of the Johns Hopkins Hospital.

Welch in an address to this society in 1892 betrayed at once the confusion in his own thought and the jarring contradiction of the two elements that made up the group. There was, he said, a "class of people who prefer squalor and darkness to decency and light, who need moral reformation before they can be properly moved into better surroundings." Sanitary reform is only one means of "elevating the condition of the poor" and other agencies, presumably the churches, "occupy a much loftier plane." But just as the conscience of the comfortable classes was dropping off to sleep, Welch broke in with another voice and thrust aside everything that he had said by questioning whether moral regeneration was possible in the circumstances in which the poorest people lived. Nevertheless, for the time being, he as the great Influential of the medical profession had given religious and moral reformers equal importance with sanitarians in helping the poor. Concessions of this sort were the condition of a vigorous Charity Organization movement.

Welch stood committed in any event to the proposition that prolonging the lives of the poor, sick, and enfeebled by outside assistance was socially desirable. The period from 1860 to 1914, through which he himself lived, encompassed almost the whole history of Social Darwinism and the substitution for the accumulated morality and ethics of mankind of the formula of the survival of the fittest. How weak the hold of Social Darwinism was at its height may be gathered from the very fact that scientific medicine under Welch's leadership took hold in America at the same time, and this in the context of the hospital with its one abiding tradition of an even-handed extension of charity to all comers. In this light the doctrine of Social Darwinism falls into perspective as an intellectual fad of short life and shallow roots.

Welch repudiated the argument that reduction of the rate of infant mortality interfered with natural selection. But he did so without making any real contact with the arguments, whatever their merit, put forward by the Social Darwinians. He let himself be carried along on a tide of indignation and humane feeling and simply by-passed any rational confrontation of the philosophy with which he was contending. In this he was merely the representative of his age. Social Darwinism collapsed against the unshakable impulse of mankind to pull as many people on to the raft of life as possible, even at the risk of everybody going short. The field of battle was not intellectual but instinctive. It did not follow from this that sanitary reform and public health had the worse case in point of logic.

Here Welch forgot to be rational. In another direction he chose to be irrational and displayed from a fresh side the functions of an Influential. In the line of direct descent the public health movement in the English-speaking world went as far back as the 1830's and had the double interest, as Welch pointed out, of owing more to humanitarians than to men of science and of being a structure of some magnitude resting on no foundation at all in terms of knowledge about the specific cause of particular diseases. For want of this knowledge the "filth theory" of disease prevailed, and the work of the sanitarian was in a perfectly literal sense to clean things up.

When Pasteur and Koch ushered in the age of bacteriology in Welch's early manhood, a genuinely scientific substructure was for the first time thrust beneath the public health movement. But the rethinking of public health policies in the light of bacteriology was painfully slow and hesitant. The chief revisionist in America, Charles V. Chapin of Providence, Rhode Island, with his open assault on the filth theory and undiscriminating cleanups, had scarcely come into his own before 1910. Yet many of his points were made in earlier writings of Welch. It was Welch, but might have been Chapin, who wrote in 1892: "We may drink contaminated water, breathe impure air and live on a polluted soil without getting typhoid or typhus fever, or diphtheria or scarlet fever or other infectious disease. These influences may be and doubtless are deleterious to health, but unless the specific germs of disease have been introduced, they do not produce well defined diseases."

Nevertheless, Welch justified the traditional public health measures. "Cleanliness and comfort demand" purification of "the ground on which we live, the air which we breathe, and the water and food with which we are supplied, and we must meet these needs without waiting to learn just what relation infectious agents bear to the earth, air, water, and food." The filth theory of disease had been a good thing. Though "incomplete and even erroneous in many respects," it indirectly reduced the death rate and led to social improvements.

A more candid statement that unsound theories can be justified by empirical results would be hard to find, or a more calculated affront to a certain form of the scientific temper, here represented by Chapin. Welch drew back almost instinctively — but quite consciously as well — from the rational public health movement commended by Chapin, in lock step with science and therefore in danger of being cut off from many ends and aspirations which it had once served. Welch deliberately strengthened the forces making for inertia in the sanitary tradition and declined to contract the horizons of the public health movement to the limits apparently imposed by bacteriology. The limits were too narrow, but Welch did not dwell on this point and clearly had something else in mind. By a calculated sacrifice of scientific rigor he hoped to quell any incipient panic among the public health workers and restore to them enough of their corporate morale to make possible a gradual assimilation of new theories. The whole episode displayed the estrangement of the Influential from the internal standards of a science which he was engaged in fitting into the pattern of society at large.

By his benevolent attitude toward the filth theory of

disease, regarded as making for a better civic life, Welch demonstrated a habit of mind that might be termed "the socialism of hygiene." The underlying philosophy as phrased by Welch's chosen successor as head of the State Board of Health of Maryland was simple. "Certain things have had to be done to give the best possible services to the people of Maryland. If they could not be done one way they had to be done another. That's all." Any political and social innovations needed to attain the maximum of public health were justified.

This pursuit, not of the minimum of decency but the maximum of well-being, took on the widest possible significance when joined to Welch's conviction that "there are no social, no industrial, no economic problems which are not related to problems of health. The better conditions of living, housing, working conditions in factories, pure food, a better supply of drinking water, all these great questions, social, industrial and economic, are bound up with the problems of public health." Whoever dealt with public health would find his scope coextensive with the life of society. He could shut his eyes to no abuse once the barrier between the immediate and the remote causes of disease was annihilated in this way.

The final ingredient of a socialism, both dilute and unconscious, was to assign the keeping of the public health to governmental agents. No fear that these agents might become too numerous or too powerful seems ever to have entered Welch's head. Though arguing for the primacy of local control, he said in 1909 that one of the greatest needs of the United States was the "extension and improvement" of a public health organization under the national government. With this object in view he had already given up in

1901 his long opposition to the Marine Hospital Service and devoted his energies to strengthening it as the only feasible nucleus of a national public health service. In 1902 the Marine Hospital Service became the United States Public Health and Marine Hospital Service. Throughout he took the position that coercive powers of greater or less magnitude must lie with some level of government, national if that were more efficient than local.

The question remained whether the socialism of hygiene was or was not to be democratic. Here Welch confronted one of the recurring dilemmas of the professional scientist, and particularly of a man like himself, the commander of an army of experts with their claim to be superior in intellect and training to the mass of the people: should the expert work upon an inert and passive people for their own benefit, but as little as possible with their active co-operation; or encourage the people, with their inexhaustible fund of — possibly dangerous — energies, to help themselves on expert advice. It was possible to argue, with Welch's former student Hermann M. Biggs, Director of Public Health in New York City, that the authoritarianism in public hygiene need not be disguised in a democracy. "We are prepared, when necessary," he said in 1897, "to introduce and enforce, and the people are ready to accept, measures which might seem radical and arbitrary, if they were not plainly designed for the public good, and evidently beneficent in their effects." Biggs thought that "more arbitrary" measures could be introduced in the United States than elsewhere "simply because our government is democratic." In this spirit Biggs undertook in 1914 to break off the tourist trade of Niagara Falls until the local authorities admitted the existence of a smallpox epidemic and instituted public vaccinations; and won his point.

Welch, for his part, was reluctant to conclude that scientific medicine in its application to daily life ought to be an enclave of authoritarianism in a democratic society. He hoped instead that it could be made a common possession and even a common enterprise of the whole body of citizens.

Thus, once the revelation had come at the beginning of the twentieth century that tuberculosis was a form of *social* pathology, an index of poverty, overwork, and ignorance, Welch and Osler took the lead in organizing laymen for the first time in history into a full-scale campaign against a particular disease. This step deserves to rank with mass conscription, the marketing of government securities to the citizens at large, and the institution of a popular press as one of the decisive events in the involvement of the whole of mankind in the making of their own history. Welch as the leader of an organized profession, with a long tradition of self-containment and secrecy, had certain misgivings. Why, he asked, was it "necessary to arouse the public regarding the prevention of tuberculosis more than concerning other preventable diseases?" His answer was that prevention of tuberculosis was a "social and economical" as well as medical problem. On these grounds Welch gave his blessing to the formation in 1904 of what later became the National Tuberculosis Association, and served as its president in 1911. The founding of other such groups followed. Welch took part in many, most conspicuously in the mental-health movement, which sprang up as the result of Clifford Beers's autobiography *A Mind That*

Found Itself of 1908, the story of a man, not a physician, who had come back from the insane.

Welch was eager to break the conspiracy of silence among laymen about insanity and other kinds of illness. In 1913 his colleague Thomas S. Cullen, Howard Kelly's collaborator in gynecology, decided that the death rate from cancer could only be cut if women learned to recognize the early symptoms and sought early treatment. Cullen and Kelly made a practice at Johns Hopkins of sending tissues from their patients to be examined for cancer in Welch's laboratory. They found much unsuspected cancer with which surgeons like themselves and Halsted could deal successfully in the early stages. Cullen, with Welch's full approval, put the question before the oracle of American women, the bachelor Edward W. Bok of *The Ladies' Home Journal*, and secured the publication of a series of articles by the muckraking journalist Samuel Hopkins Adams in the *Journal* for 1913, "What Can We Do About Cancer?"

Welch had gone far by the standards of his time in enlisting the aid of the public and giving to the public health movement a democratic and permissive tinge. But in one critical matter he hesitated to call the people into action — in defense of vivisection and animal experimentation. In this one region alone he had found part of the people already fighting on the wrong side at the beginning of his career.

Welch had said of the public health movement that it owed more to humanitarians than medical men. He now had to deal with the nightmare humanitarians of antivivisection, where the impulse that cleaned up the cities and succored the poor had turned dark, sour, and cunning; the exasperated revenge of mankind upon itself for having put down the rubbish of the ages and founded scientific medicine. Welch was left looking at the other side of the paintings of Sir Edwin Landseer: a raising of cats, dogs, and horses not to the level of men but above men.

The whole movement had sprung up well within Welch's own lifetime. The classic exposition of antivivisection, by the English veterinary surgeon George Fleming, dated from 1864. Fleming was never surpassed for scurrility and illogic in a swelling literature of shrill untruth. He called the vivisectionist "a remorseless inquisitor, who attempts to wring the secrets of nature from his victims by the most harrowing and protracted tortures"; worse than "the hangman, the headsman, and the butcher." Fleming proposed, as a few others had already done, that no experiments should be performed except in the presence of a "jury" of observers. But he concluded by saying that animal experimentation was in fact totally unnecessary, "confusing and prolific of error."

In the early 1870's a number of incidents aroused public opinion in England and led to the passage in 1876 of an act requiring investigators to secure a license from the Home Secretary for each research involving vivisection. This measure, which forced men like Lister to work from time to time in foreign laboratories, touched off efforts at similar legislation in America.

The effectual founder in the United States of antivivisection was Henry Bergh, a lean lank-haired Puritan, who created in 1864 an American Society for the Prevention of Cruelty to Animals on the model of the British group. For a time his efforts did not conflict and even coincided with those of the sanitary reformers, whom he helped in cleaning up the dairy industry of New York City. But in 1879, under the stimulus supplied by Parliament, he led a movement in New York State to secure total prohibition of all animal experimentation. Bergh's reckless misrepresentations on this occasion backfired and the measure failed.

By this time a network of antivivisection had spread across the Western world. In Germany the most effective spokesman was Ernst von Weber, author of *The Torture-Chambers of Science* of 1879, with its drawing "from the life" of a dog with pipe in mouth and a glass of beer before it and the appended question, "Should animals like this be cut up alive?" The leader in England was now Frances Power Cobbe, who published in 1892 her famous book *The Nine Circles, or the Hell of the Innocent Described from the Reports of the Presiding Spirits*, with its misrepresentation of the work of the great brain surgeon Sir Victor Horsley. In the United States the physician Albert Leffingwell was perhaps the most conspicuous of a large group.

When therefore Welch began his reign as an Influential, antivivisection was deeply intrenched: a world alliance of overlapping animal lovers, vegetarians, anti-Listerians, antibacteriologists, and anti-inoculationists; soft muddleheaded women, cold-blooded Amazons and publicity seekers of both sexes, bluff advocates of the old-fashioned godliness and soap-and-water but not carbolic-acid cleanliness, maudlin religionists not averse to blasphemy, medical sectaries, and academic and professional castoffs — all engaged in a travesty of the intellectual life, snooping about laboratories and ransacking the pages of scientific journals for ammunition.

In the mid-nineties, however, the antivivisectionists of the United States had not yet secured from any state the restrictive legislation which they were willing to accept for the moment in lieu of total prohibition. They then adopted the traditional strategy of attempting to break the log jam by inducing Congress to take a pattern stand in legislation for the District of Columbia. In this spirit the antivivisectionists turned to the homeopathic physician who was chairman of the Senate Committee on the District, Senator Jacob H. Gallinger, of New Hampshire.

From 1896 forward he introduced at their behest numerous variants of a single measure. The core of his proposals was a scheme for licensing individual pieces of research, with detailed reports as to the outcome and the free entry into all laboratories of outside observers likely to be from their mode of choice antivivisectionists. Serious restrictions were placed on the anesthetic agents to be used and the possibility of allowing an animal to recover and emerge from the anesthetic was severely hedged about. In the grant of licenses, the test was laid down that the projected researches should promise some clear benefit to be stated in advance. At one time Gallinger's bill also forbade a human being to consent to an experiment upon himself likely to put his life in danger. This provision, if applied, as Congress had the right to apply it, to members of the armed services, would shortly have prevented Walter Reed from demonstrating the mode of transmission of yellow fever.

In 1896 on the first occasion when Gallinger got his

bill reported out of committee — unanimously — Welch drew up a resolution of protest from the Association of American Physicians; went with Osler to Washington to put pressure on Senator Arthur P. Gorman of Maryland; enlisted the aid of a classmate at Yale, Senator Edward O. Wolcott of Colorado; and kept the measure from reaching the floor of the Senate. In 1897 Welch again responded to the challenge as a politician of great skill and spent most of the winter whipping his forces into line. He dined out in political society with the help of the Baltimore hostesses and guided conversation into the proper channel, stimulated dozens of organizations into passing appropriate resolutions, asked the private physicians of all the senators to write personal notes to their patients, and went himself from senator to senator seeking pledges. He secured about forty, and Mark Hanna told him the bill would not be pushed. When Welch finally descended on Washington in February 1898, the battle had already been won, at least for the moment. But he had to take a leading role, though less strenuous, in fending off fresh attempts by Gallinger in 1900 and 1902 to slip some kind of restrictive legislation through the Senate.

Many of the points made by Welch on these occasions were obvious: the reliance of physiology and pathology on animal experimentation from the time of Harvey forward; the unprecedented medical advances of the nineteenth century, largely as a result of vivisection; the care taken by investigators to cause no more pain than necessary; the absence even of alleged abuses in America; and the perversion of humane feeling into "inhumanity" by ignorant fanatics. But he fixed in particular on the licensing process and the conditioning of a license on prior proof that the research in question would be useful. He had long realized that "the most important discoveries in science, come not from those who make utility their guiding principle, but from the investigators of truth for its own sake." "It is impossible to foresee what may be the practical application tomorrow of any pathological fact discovered in the laboratory, no matter how remote from practical bearing it may seem today."

Now narrow utilitarianism was to be sanctioned by law, and administered by lay politicians or general practitioners, who were sure to compound the shortsightedness of the law itself. The whole process of the self-government of science by which Welch had been raised up from among the scientists themselves to make policy and guide the course of research was threatened. He might have wished in some kind of dream world to leave off being an Influential and go back to the laboratory; but the sacrifice having been made, he could not allow outsiders to play the role that had fallen to him. Under a system of licensing animal experimentation, he said, "Not those who know, but those who do not know would be given a discretion which might prove disastrous to the future of scientific medicine." He saw the whole antivivisection movement as an effort to reverse the outcome of the age-old battle for "freedom of investigation."

Welch had beaten Gallinger by an essentially private operation which brought expert opinion directly to bear on the legislators. When in 1908 the physiologist Walter B. Cannon of Harvard called for a joint group of laymen and physicians in defense of medical research, Welch had grave misgivings. A counterorganization of this kind, he wrote, would be an open acknowledgment of the strength of the antivivisectionists. Laymen were likely to see no harm in mild restrictive measures and to insist on concessions of which there would be no end once begun; and besides he himself had shown that the problem could be dealt with otherwise. Cannon was a rising man, but Welch was and remained the great Influential. By contrast with England, no lay group in support of vivisection was then formed in America. In this matter, Welch never learned to trust the mass of the people.

Thus he as an Influential cut across all living and vigorous philosophies of society and the state: Social Darwinism, socialism, democracy. Every great movement of social thought and reform in his time was reflected in his own work, but none made him a prisoner. He always remained large-minded, tolerant, and undogmatic.

XI
The Rockefeller Institute

THE IDEA of government support for research in the universities, as distinguished from the work of the Department of Agriculture and the Public Health Service, did not enter into Welch's plans. Indeed, by its absence it went to define his place in the succession of Influentials. The new source of income, which he more than anyone else had to pass upon, was not the government but the millionaire. He now had to develop concrete policies for laboratories brought into being by lay philanthropists and cut off from any direct contact with the universities.

By the most favorable accounts, the elder Rockefeller had not found in the conduct of his business much occasion for the ethical life. But he was a Baptist, and not a hypocrite; and the displaced conscience was bound to exacerbate itself into unprecedented exertions elsewhere.

The fact that much of his money went in the end to medicine sprang from the spare-time reading of Frederick T. Gates. Gates, a handsome man with a thick head of hair, a large mustache, small shrewd eyes and a flickering smile, was a Baptist clergyman who had come to be the externalized conscience of the Rockefellers and the old man's

THE ROCKEFELLER INSTITUTE 153

chief adviser in philanthropic matters. Gates had taken as his work in life the task of seeing that the whole family was not damned to eternity by the reproach of hoarding up money to no better end than being wealthy. In 1897 he read Osler's *Principles and Practice of Medicine*. Osler was a "therapeutic nihilist" who left no doubt in the mind of an intelligent reader — and Gates was highly intelligent — that almost nothing was yet known about the specific cure of specific diseases. Gates saw at once an opportunity to put the Rockefeller money to work. At a time when dogmatic theology had already begun to sink toward its low-water mark in America, Gates as a clergyman persuaded himself that scientific medicine was a kind of theological research. Many years later he described the Rockefeller Institute to an audience of scientists as a "theological seminary." "Why do you laugh?" he said. "I am now talking about the religion, not of the past, but of the future, and I tell you that as this medical research goes on you will . . . promulgate . . . new moral laws and new social laws, new definitions of what is right and wrong in our relations with each other." "You will teach nobler conceptions of our social relations and of the God who is over us all."

In the spirit of this accommodation of religion to science on the terms of science, Gates drew up a memorandum for the elder Rockefeller — and waited patiently. He knew from experience that the old man did not like to be nudged and could not be hurried. The younger Rockefeller, with whom Gates chiefly dealt, was favorable from the beginning, but not till the spring of 1901 was he ready to make a decisive move on behalf of his father. He then asked the lawyer Starr J. Murphy, Gates, Dr. L. Emmett

Holt, of New York, and Dr. Christian A. Herter, Welch's student, to form a group of medical advisers on the establishment of an independent institution for medical research.

Welch was brought in at once by common consent, with his friend T. Mitchell Prudden, of Physicians and Surgeons, and his former student, now head of the New York City board of health, Hermann M. Biggs. Welch became chairman of the advisory board, and from this time forward he was the leader of the whole enterprise. Any other response would seriously have diminished his stature as the chief Influential of the biological sciences. Yet he had certain misgivings, notably because there was no university connection. He feared "that in the zeal for the promotion of scientific investigation by the endowment of independent institutions, sight should be lost of the ultimate dependence of such investigation upon educational conditions. The supply of trained workers must come from the colleges and universities." But his effort in 1901 to forge some kind of link between the new institution and Columbia University was put down with great firmness by the Rockefellers and their advisers; and Welch knew better than to insist. He therefore made the best he could of the situation. With his deep commitment to the university ideal, he had the ironic task of recreating within independent rival institutions enough of the university spirit to make them serious competitors of Harvard, Columbia, Chicago — and Johns Hopkins. He had to share out the university tone and aura and make less distinctive the tradition which it had been the work of his life to build. What had to be done he did.

In May 1901 the other members of the advisory board

authorized Welch to offer the directorship of the new institute to the great animal pathologist Theobald Smith. When Smith refused, Welch supervised the congenial task of dividing the sum of $26,450, for the years 1901 and 1902 combined, among a surprisingly large number of research men in the universities. One of the recipients was apprehensive lest the subsidies lead to a glutting of the market for medical scientists.

In January 1902 Welch wrote to Rockefeller, Jr. to say that an independent laboratory ought now to be established, and early in March his favorite pupil, Simon Flexner, agreed to take the directorship. Flexner, who was doing a brilliant job at the University of Pennsylvania, had hesitated for a time to come into an enterprise which had as yet no guarantee of permanence. He yielded when Welch told him, "Flexner, they will never desert you." In June of the same year the elder Rockefeller, on the suggestion of his son, pledged $1,000,000 to be expended over a period of ten years. After a last year of grants in 1903, the temporary laboratories of the Rockefeller Institute — so named at the urging of Welch and the other advisers — were opened in 1904. In 1906 the official laboratory building was dedicated with an address by Welch on "The Benefits of the Endowment of Medical Research." Finally, in November 1907, Rockefeller instituted a permanent endowment — initially of $2,620,610.

Welch now made the one serious slip of his career as an Influential. The affairs of the institute were divided between the trustees (including Gates, Murphy, and Rockefeller, Jr.), who held the funds, and the Board of Scientific Directors (including Welch, Herter, Holt, Prudden, Biggs, Smith, and Flexner), who passed upon the researches. But

Welch proposed in 1906 that the trustees should have the right of approving the annual budget and any special outlays not included in the budget. Herter and others protested strongly and prevailed. Though the trustees were then men of judgment, character, and humility, Welch's proposal would have allowed persons outside the scientific community to intrude upon the self-government of science. This, as he had never before failed to see, was fundamentally wrong and destructive of the meaning of his own career. Another of his proposals made in 1906, the rendering of reports by the trustees and directors to each other, was adopted at once and led to the famous scientific reports of later years.

Though Welch worked hard to make the Rockefeller Institute a success, he continued to regard the university as the true home of research. He therefore made the most of a request from the Rockefellers in 1907 that the scientific directors offer an opinion on the advisability of helping the medical school of McGill University, which had just been struck by fire. Welch at once converted this limited inquiry into a recommendation that Rockefeller make large-scale benefactions to medical schools in general, on the one condition that they approximate to the standards of Johns Hopkins and Harvard. No response was made to the proposal at the time, and no money given to McGill.

Welch continued as president of the Scientific Directors till 1933, and remained through the whole period of his service the member with the best grasp of the most things. But he made his unique contribution at the beginning — partly in the form of personnel like Simon Flexner, partly in the form of standards, partly in the form of giving to

THE ROCKEFELLER INSTITUTE 157

the whole enterprise the certificate of good character that only he could supply.

Pressure from the Rockefellers for practical results he did not encounter. As Gates later said, ". . . we did not cherish extravagant dreams." He and the Rockefellers had agreed that no important discoveries were likely to flow from the Rockefeller Institute itself; but that they might set an example for other wealthy men, and perhaps contribute to the making of discoveries elsewhere. When Rockefeller, Jr. learned in 1902 that some valuable results had been obtained by the recipients of a grant-in-aid from the institute, he wrote at once to tell Welch that this success was "far more important than we could have hoped for so soon." Short-term utilitarianism and the promise of quick results would not have gratified the Rockefellers. Welch could afford to move cautiously and promise nothing. In the end he got word from the family that none of the Rockefeller benefactions had been as well managed as the institute. The feeling of peace of mind about the work of the institute which Welch more than anyone else gave to the Rockefellers may possibly have been his most important contribution and the ultimate cause of the larger and larger gifts that eventually came to the institute.

The Carnegie Institution of Washington was the counterpart for the physical sciences of the Rockefeller Institute for the biological. Welch became a trustee of the Carnegie Institution in 1906, after the formative period under Daniel C. Gilman was well begun, and chairman of the executive committee in 1909. He remained as chairman till 1916 and died a trustee in 1934. For some seven or eight years he was therefore head of the advisory board of both of the leading research foundations in America, the greatest Influential of medicine and biology and a leading figure in the physical sciences as well.

With the possible exception of Benjamin Franklin, no one had ever occupied a more central place in the life of science in America. But Welch as a human being led a life of quiet desperation and desperate fortitude, torn in a thousand directions by a thousand solicitations. Of the few people with whom he might have been glad to share his triumphs, his father died in 1892, his stepmother Emily Welch in 1901, his brother-in-law Stuart Walcott in 1905, and his sister Emma in 1910. Apart from his colleagues at the Hopkins, he made one close friend in Baltimore, the fabulous Major Richard M. Venable. Venable, a bachelor with an enormous paunch, was a gourmet, a woman-hater, a free-thinker, and a gentleman politician who ruled Baltimore from behind the scenes — but not very far behind. He too died as early as 1910. The man who most nearly filled his place in later years was Alfred Jenkins Shriver, like Venable a lawyer and a bachelor.

Meanwhile Welch tried to keep from drowning in a flood of paper — great quantities of letters and journals and articles flowing in from day to day without end, thrown on the desk and there layered off from time to time by an outspread newspaper, heaped in crazy mountains on the chairs, piled up and falling over on the floor, thrust frantically onto shelves, fighting back malevolently and contending with Welch for mastery. In all of this he tried to think that there was system of a kind. When Hugh Young called and found eight chairs full of unopened mail, Welch protested that there was no real disorder. "On that armchair there I have the letters that have come during the past week; I hope to read these in the near future. On that chair I have the letters that have come within the past month. On the other chairs are letters and magazines anywhere from six months to a year old which I hope to get to sometime." On the desk Young counted four layers bounded by their newspapers. In his prime Welch never had a secretary, scorned the proffer of mechanical devices like the dictaphone, and never did catch up with his mail. In time the friends who had been horrified by a glimpse into his study came to realize that no one had ever heard of a letter of the first importance that did not get a prompt reply.

In one direction Welch fell further and further behind. One perquisite of every great Influential had come to be possession of a scholarly journal, and Welch founded in 1896 a much-needed *Journal of Experimental Medicine*. In a short time contributors began to find that their manuscripts had been swallowed up into some kind of abyss and were never heard from again. Frantic letters asking for the return of the article for publication elsewhere met with no response. Hurd would sometimes scavenge through Welch's study and retrieve a manuscript — in Welch's absence — but the situation rapidly became hopeless. In the end, to Welch's great relief, possession of the *Journal* passed from Johns Hopkins to the Rockefeller Institute in 1904.

From this continual nightmare of more things to do than he had time for, Welch found such respite as he could — with Venable and Shriver at the Maryland and University Clubs, with his landlady's young daughter whom he liked to talk to for a few minutes late at night, by himself on weekends at Atlantic City. He told his sister that he liked his resorts "vulgar." These unexplained departures from Baltimore led to much ribald conjecture among the medical students.

> Nobody knows where Popsy eats,
> Nobody knows where Popsy sleeps,
> Nobody knows whom Popsy keeps,
>   But Popsy.

His only vices seem in fact to have been gorging on desserts and riding the roller coaster.

One way and another Welch kept up his courage and lived in the midst of his papers and did his work as well as he could. As a reward he kept his vision and sense of perspective uncorrupted to the end. At the great testimonial dinner in Baltimore in 1910, with 500 guests, to celebrate his being president of the American Medical Association, he still spoke of the Influential's business, into which he had been drawn so many years before, as "outside work" and tried against the grain of the occasion to record his own sense of failure and division within himself. "I cannot but regret," he said, "a certain amount of dissipation of energy," and he warned the younger men present to "guard against taking up so many different things as I have undertaken." Here his audience had begun to stir uneasily, and he made the last sacrifice of covering over the truth which he had begun to speak and went on with a funny story to tell of the satisfactions which he had had. He could not let his hearers down; but for himself he would always belong to the unself-deceived.

XII
Osler and After Osler

Though Welch swung out in wider and wider loops, Johns Hopkins was the immovable center of his world. In 1900 he might have been excused for thinking that the fabric of the Hopkins had been built to last out his time. All the chief figures in the medical faculty might hope to live for another twenty years or more, and all of them together had fallen into a kind of habit of success. They need only not break their stride to go on from triumph to triumph. But the mixture was unstable and a crisis approached. The key figures were Welch, Mall, and Osler, and Mall above the others.

Mall was the greatest American anatomist and by far the most distinguished scientist on the medical faculty — the strongest link in the creative tradition. A small trim handsome man, unhurried with his single experiment each day, a perfectionist in all of his undertakings — and almost perfect — quiet, sarcastic, self-effacing, and inexorable, he was the man of iron will who wore down opposing wills and always had his way. He was feared by most students when they were under his control and thereafter hated by some with a hatred that was not appeased by his death and still breaks out after fifty years.

His "inductive method" of teaching anatomy to beginners, by which he meant giving them something to cut with and something to cut and going away and leaving them alone, left the student ignorant of regional anatomy and forced the surgeons to offer instruction of their own. "Mall failed the men." But this kind of failure he prided himself upon as setting anatomy free from its old subservience to medicine. He meant to be a man of science and a teacher of scientists, who would have to make their own accommodation to practical medicine. The operative word in scientific medicine was for him "scientific." It was no accident that Gertrude Stein, who was good at science but had no vocation for medicine, preferred Mall to all of her other instructors at Johns Hopkins. Nor was it any accident that he succeeded brilliantly with advanced students and created a school of anatomists of equal importance with the Welch school of pathology. And by these students he was idolized, as by Gertrude Stein, for whom he ranked with William James among the academic men of her acquaintance for sharpness of outline, bite, flavor, and insight.

Mall did not meet with uniform hostility from the clinical men, who had to make in the first instance not scientists but physicians. The chief surgeon of the Johns Hopkins Hospital happened above every other surgeon of his time in America to belong to the laboratory tradition; and apart from Welch, Mall was Halsted's best friend. One of Halsted's chief pleasures was to talk with Mall about current and projected researches. Mall could be sure of never being reproached by Halsted for being a poor teacher. One could almost say that Mall's best work was Halsted.

This identification was well understood at the time, and by no one better than Osler, whom it maddened, baffled, and frightened to see a great surgeon warped from medicine to science, so that one of the clinical professors had gone over to the enemy. Osler never attempted to conceal his distaste for the "inductive method" of teaching anatomy, and he always deplored in private the remoteness of Mall and Halsted from the students and their elevation of research above teaching and science above medicine. "A man who is not fond of students and who does not suffer their foibles gladly," he wrote, "misses the greatest zest in life; and the teacher who wraps himself in the cloak of his researches, and lives apart from the bright spirits of the coming generation, is very apt to find his garment the shirt of Nessus." The public, he said, would insist that scholars in any institution founded for the advancement of medicine devote themselves to the cure of disease and the prevention of death; and the public was right.

Every item in this indictment fitted either Mall or Halsted or both. But when all three men were colleagues together the lines of battle were never clearly drawn; and except for the open scandal of the "inductive method," Osler and Mall engaged in no real controversies. But personalities maneuvering for conflict will make themselves felt in advance of the appropriate issue. At Johns Hopkins there was a gradual clearing up of the relationship of Mall to Welch as seen through Osler's eyes, a kind of shaping up of the human situation that no one could lay hold of with any assurance till everything burst into the open and cast light behind it.

Mall was said to teach, if at all, not by guiding the hand

but jogging the elbow and looking in with a word of advice from time to time; and his enemies liked to think of his role at the Hopkins in these terms — "gumshoe tactics" with no speeches, but a quiet suggestion from behind someone else's shoulder, and a whispered question for someone else to put, and a murmur of deprecation at the wrong answer. His friends and admirers painted the same portrait of a man of enormous self-assurance but no stage presence. At the beginning of the twentieth century many people felt certain that Mall was exercising great influence over Welch from behind the scenes.

Mall had, in the nature of things, an unshakable hold on Welch. He had been the most difficult of the whole medical faculty to secure for Johns Hopkins, and could at any time have gone elsewhere, as to Harvard in 1912; and the fact of his coming was almost entirely a tribute to Welch. But at a much deeper level Mall represented for Welch the ideal of the scientific life: an unbroken line of researches from youth into age, with no distractions or diversions, the perfect embodiment of the creative tradition, the man whom Welch would himself have wished to be.

If Welch had been a smaller man of the kind who as he ceases to live up to his own ideals begins to think that they were not worthy of him, the result would certainly have been an ever-increasing estrangement of Mall and himself. But the perfection and integrity, in both senses of the term, of his career lay precisely in remaining faithful to his first ideals and rejoicing to see them fulfilled by others if not himself. Given this fact, Welch could not have done otherwise than defer to Mall on what both of them regarded as the central issues of academic life — the pre-eminence of research and the unity of good scholarship and good teaching. There is an almost placating note in a letter written by Welch to Mall in 1893: "I agree with you in begrudging time spent by men whose capacity is for scientific investigation in organizing and in executive work, although we shall have a great deal of this to do." The more Welch departed from Mall's standard — and his own — of the right expenditure of time, the more Mall gained in moral supremacy over him.

The issue that made this seem a matter of critical importance was "full-time." In the winter of 1885–1886 when Mall was working with Carl Ludwig in Leipzig, the old man had confided to him one last dream, of placing clinical medicine on a university basis, with the clinical professors, as well as the preclinical, devoting their full time to research rather than engaging in private practice on the side. This idea Mall had taken with him to the University of Chicago, where it seems already to have been making headway before his arrival. After Mall returned to Baltimore, he worked closely with the Canadian Lewellys F. Barker, who had studied with Welch before the opening of the medical school. In due time Barker went to Chicago to fill Mall's old chair. From this vantage point he delivered in 1902 a famous address to the Western alumni of Johns Hopkins in which he came out for clinical full-time and attracted general attention throughout the country. He made no secret of having been influenced by Mall.

From this time forward full-time threatened to split the medical profession in two. If the experiment were to have any prospect of success it would need the prestige of the best medical school in America behind it. But nothing could be done without winning over one or the other of the two great charismatic figures of the Hopkins faculty; and if Welch and Osler took up opposite positions there would sooner or later be a confrontation of personalities and ideals from which the medical school might never recover. Osler, a clinician with a large private practice, was from the beginning utterly opposed to the whole idea for the same reasons that he feared and mistrusted its sponsor Mall as a doctrinaire of pure science. The unknown in the situation was Welch.

During Osler's time in Baltimore Welch made only one short address on the teaching of clinical medicine, in 1901. He then called for advanced training in clinical research and spoke of the need for recruiting clinical as well as preclinical professors from the country at large. This step would discard success in local practice as the test of fitness for a chair. But it did not follow that clinical men chosen for their bent toward research would choose not to engage in practice. The best of them might be expected like Osler and Kelly to become consultants and surgeons in great local demand. Welch had not yet gone the whole way with Mall.

That he would end, however, by going beyond this point was predetermined by everything that he had done and been and Osler had not; and beneath the surface if not above there would have to be a final definition of the antithesis between them. For Mall could only exert influence upon Welch, who was neither weak nor pliable, on the condition of their being at bottom the same kind of man. Consciously or not, those, like Osler, who feared Mall were ultimately fearful of Welch himself; and in this they were right.

Full-time was said by its enemies to be an untried experiment which might fail. But so had been the life-pattern of Welch; and so also had been the whole conception of the Johns Hopkins University, Hospital, and Medical School. Welch had always struck out for the unoccupied territory, and he had never yet been disappointed.

Full-time was said by its enemies to be doctrinaire and impractical. But to study in Germany rather than to go home to Norfolk had been impractical; to go from New York to Baltimore had been in Fred Dennis's opinion "impractical"; to require a college degree, with French and German, for entrance to a medical school had been doctrinaire in the extreme. In retrospect Welch's own specialty had been to make the things that would not work, work.

Full-time was said, finally, to be depersonalizing and destructive of human relationships. Full-time men, so the argument ran, would be isolated and cut off from the local profession, both from the nature of their work and the kind of temperament that would be likely to take it up — scientific, self-contained, and a little cold. But Welch too had deliberately cut himself off from the work of a consultant and by so much diminished the range of his acquaintances. And he preserved an inviolable remoteness, of a pleasant sort, from all but a handful of men. His own popularity served to conceal the significance of the fact that the two members of the medical faculty whom he had been most conspicuous in bringing to Baltimore were Halsted and Mall — the least popular of the instructors, the most withdrawn from living contacts, the most doctrinaire in their commitment to science as opposed to medical empiricism. They were, in fact, precisely the men in whom Osler found and feared the image of the "full-time man."

For Welch their intellectual distinction predominated over any possible defects, and this was for him a general principle in academic appointments — "perhaps we attach too much importance to personality versus scholarly achievement." The roots of this de-emphasizing of personality went deep into Welch's own character and temperament, and were largely independent of circumstances. But perhaps his role of Influential had strengthened a native impulse to judge men of science not by their qualities of personal address but by their intellects. For it may well have been the condition of maintaining his self-respect, as he withdrew from the research enterprise, to go on sharing with the productive scientists their emphasis on intellectual capacity above everything else. He had become a kind of politician in the cause of science; but he was incapable of being merely a politician, who valued the political arts for their own sake. If the coming of full-time were to mean that in the filling of clinical chairs a man's personality would only count in so far as he knew how to project it through the medium of his research, this would be for Welch not a loss but an incalculable gain.

Osler, who had done research and introduced important innovations in teaching and administration, was the last man whom Welch would have charged with trading upon his personality. If Osler had been gruff, secretive, and unforthcoming as a human being, he would still have left a mark on the history of medicine. But it was for personal qualities and unmediated disclosures of himself that men loved and followed Osler in life and after death; and he for his part had almost a mystique of personality and warm human relationships. He was and meant to be an ethical figure, who saw in medicine not only a means of healing the sick but of giving "unity, peace, and concord" to the healers. For him it was left to speak of the local medical society in the same tone that other men had reserved for the regiment and the congregation — a place where all selfish wills must be yielded up and animosities put aside. For a man who consistently struck this note, full-time was a moral calamity, a disastrous impoverishment of the clinical man's right and duty to be implicated in the whole community of physicians. A man who stood aside from the process of humanizing and being humanized by the friction of personal contacts might be a scientist but never a doctor. The increasing application of science to medicine left Osler unshaken in his conviction that medicine itself must remain an art and distinctively the art of establishing personal rapport between the physician and the patient.

At Johns Hopkins, Osler was balanced for a time against Welch. But no balance of which Osler was a term could endure for very long. It was in his nature always to be moving on. As early as 1894 Howard Kelly had told Tom Cullen that Osler wanted to go to England and be knighted; and the opportunity to take the first step came in 1904 with the offer of the Regius Professorship of Medicine at Oxford. Osler was then tired, overwhelmed by his responsibilities in America, and conscious of having done the work which he had meant to do at the Hopkins.

Yet his prompt acceptance of the chair at Oxford went much deeper than this, and deeper still than the desire to live in England and send his son to an English school and have a title. In his farewell address at Johns Hopkins in February 1905 he attributed the success of the university in great part to "the concentration of a group of light-horse intellectuals, without local ties." When academic men began to be wedded to one place and one institution for life they ceased to be fully alive, and university presidents ought to welcome a "nomadic spirit" in their faculties.

He who had made almost a philosophy of close human relationships tore himself up by the roots not once but three times and left his friends behind. He knew that he had the power to go among strangers and become part of them and make them better friends among themselves; and he wished from time to time, perhaps unconsciously, to make some fresh display of this power, to give it the maximum play, and have the sense of its being renewed in him like some gift or faculty which might have slipped away without being noticed. For such a man, coming and going might seem to be the chief business of life, both for their challenge to himself and the public occasions to which they led. No situation could have been more congenial to him than the succession of farewell dinners and meetings in his honor in 1905. He then had the opportunity to tell large groups of physicians what they had accomplished in his time by working together and the license to project without any disguise his ethic of "unity, peace, and concord" among themselves. Moreover, he had in a sense to go away from Baltimore to test the force of the impression that he had made. He had come to stand for a way of life, for ethical and moral values, and until he went away no one could be sure whether he had communicated these values to others for the term of their natural lives, or had merely imposed his own standards upon them from the outside by an act of the will from day to day; whether he had been an instrument of regeneration or merely of discipline. But if only the latter, he had failed; and the test was to go away.

Welch on hearing the news of Osler's resignation wrote that the loss would be "irreparable." But in spite of the perfect good feeling and mutual respect that always prevailed between Welch and Osler, Osler was apprehensive about the future. At the close of his last faculty meeting, he turned to Mall and said, "Now I go, and you have your way." This amounted to saying that Welch would come down in the end on the side of all the things that Osler mistrusted and feared in Mall. For Welch would now be more than ever the dominant figure in the medical school; and only through him could Mall "have his way."

Welch at fifty-five now confronted the necessity of taking hold at the Hopkins as he had not had to do since the very beginning. He had the advantage of the fact that he, not Osler, was the one indispensable man on whom everything turned. Osler's departure was shattering; the departure of Welch would have been catastrophic. But short of his own death, the loss of Osler was the most serious imaginable blow and might conceivably have broken the Hopkins stride forever. To prevent this Welch had to undertake a kind of refounding, rethinking, and reinvigoration of the medical tradition at Johns Hopkins.

His first task was to find a successor for Osler, in the knowledge that any choice would be a disappointment. Welch followed the only possible course of choosing a man who made no pretense of having the personal qualities of Osler, the tall, thin, handsome gray ascetic Lewellys F. Barker. Osler had helped to train Barker and thought highly of him. But of all possible candidates for the chair of medicine, Barker was most closely associated with Mall and full-time.

Barker was not however appointed on full-time. The innovation connected with his return to Baltimore was noncontroversial — the setting up between 1905 and 1907 of three clinical laboratories for advanced research in biology, physiology, and biochemistry. This was a distinct advance over the teaching laboratories established by Osler and was soon imitated in progressive schools throughout the country. Barker had taught anatomy at Chicago, and many pitied him as he sat hour after hour in the library working up the subject which he was going to teach in succession to the most famous clinician in the English-speaking world. He ended by gaining general respect. Welch had got successfully over the first hurdle in his task of consolidating the reputation of the medical school. Ironically, Barker came to be an enormously successful private consultant and formed the local ties desired by Osler.

Barker wished to strengthen the curriculum on the side of psychiatry, but the expense was prohibitive. In 1908, however, Clifford Beers's *A Mind That Found Itself* attracted Welch to the mental hygiene movement. In the spring of the same year, after he began to be full of the subject, he happened to talk with the millionaire philanthropist Henry Phipps about the problem of caring for the insane. Welch spoke casually and with no ulterior motive. To his surprise he shortly received a letter from Phipps saying that he would like to endow psychiatric work at Johns Hopkins. By June all the arrangements were complete. A separate building for psychiatric patients was built on the hospital grounds and the great psychiatrist

Adolf Meyer, who had helped Beers with his book, came to Baltimore as first director of the Phipps Clinic. Once again Welch without Osler had strengthened the clinical instruction.

In all of this there was nothing to which Osler himself could object; and no indication that Mall had got the upper hand. But the initiative in the development of the medical school was about to be taken from Welch by a layman, and handed over to Mall.

The layman was Simon Flexner's brother Abraham, like him another small fine-featured man, who had taken his bachelor's degree at Johns Hopkins in Gilman's prime. In many ways Gilman remained his chief inspiration forever afterward; and Flexner with his perfect sympathy for Gilman's ideals became the most intelligently loyal alumnus the university ever had. At the end of 1908 he joined the Carnegie Foundation for the Advancement of Teaching to prepare a report on medical education in the United States. For this purpose he made a great historic tour of discovery and saw for himself, unannounced, almost every medical school in America — opened the door marked "LIBRARY" at the College of Physicians and Surgeons of Los Angeles and looked in vain for books, saw the floor of the "dissecting room" at Kansas Medical College in Topeka strewn with corn "and other things" and doubling for a chicken yard, found the "laboratory" of bacteriology, pathology, and histology at Maryland Medical College in Baltimore compressed together into a few dirty test-tubes standing in pans and cigar boxes; and discovered that these and like conditions were not exceptional but the rule. Almost everywhere the faculty consisted of busy practitioners with no time for teaching well and no thought of research; few schools had control of a hospital for adequate clinical instruction; and the highest pretense to admission standards that most of them made was to require a high-school diploma or its equivalent in their catalogue and then to admit anyone who turned up.

Flexner found only one medical school in America of which he had no serious criticism, that built by his idol Gilman and his brother Simon's idol Welch. In the famous Bulletin Number Four of the Carnegie Foundation, *Medical Education in the United States and Canada,* published in 1910, Flexner proposed two chief things, that most of the medical schools should die or be killed and that the survivors should remake themselves on the pattern of Johns Hopkins. Bulletin Number Four amounted to a sentence of execution for at least half the American medical schools. Through Abraham Flexner, who did to death more bad schools in less time than any other man in the history of the world, Johns Hopkins forced all other medical schools to approximate to its own standard or die. With this historic proclamation of the supremacy of the Hopkins, one period in the life of the medical school came to an end, when Welch and Osler had pulled together. For both of the Flexners the mainspring of the whole enterprise had been Welch and Welch alone.

As a result of the success of Bulletin Number Four, Flexner went abroad in 1910 to study medical education in Europe. He spent much time in Munich and there had "an extraordinary piece of good luck." "Professor Mall of the Johns Hopkins was there with his family during the entire time." They went together to laboratories, clinics, and lectures, and Mall took Flexner in hand in his own particular way. "Lightly, almost unconsciously, he would ask the simple question which would call my attention to something which, as he thought, I ought to notice." "In the report which I subsequently wrote the chapters dealing with medical education in Germany were profoundly influenced by Mall's apparently unconscious comments, criticisms, and suggestions. He never tried to tell me anything, but led me to see what I might otherwise well have overlooked." With mature men and women of superior intelligence Mall never failed to bring off his chosen trick of teaching without teaching; and Flexner was a very important pupil.

How important only appeared when he received a summons from Frederick T. Gates, the philanthropic adviser of the Rockefellers. Gates had the most compelling of all human questions to put: What would Flexner do with a million dollars? The answer came back without hesitation. "I should give it to Dr. Welch." Why? Because with an endowment of $400,000 Welch had built "the one ideal medical school in America" as far as it went. "Think what he might do if he had a million more." Gates thereupon commissioned Flexner to prepare a report on the needs of the Hopkins.

Welch, interested but "not excited," arranged a dinner for Flexner at the Maryland Club with Mall and Halsted, and repeated the million-dollar question. After twenty years Mall's moment had come. "If," Flexner reports him as saying, "the school could get a sum of approximately a million dollars, in my judgment, there is only one thing that we ought to do with it — use every penny of its income for the purpose of placing upon a salary basis the heads and assistants in the leading clinical departments, doing for them what the school did for the underlying medical sciences when it was started. That is the great reform which needs now to be carried through." The clinical men had done brilliant work as it was; but they could do still better with full-time. Halsted, a full-time man by nature, agreed.

The issue was joined at last. At the end of a three weeks' stay in Baltimore, Flexner proposed to Gates that a million and a half dollars be given to Johns Hopkins to establish the medical, surgical, obstetrical, and pediatric clinics on the full-time basis. On receipt of Flexner's report, the General Education Board — the Rockefeller organization for such purposes — began at once to make plans for an appropriation in excess of a million dollars and awaited a request from the university.

As always everything at the medical school turned on Welch, and the question became whether he would or would not push full-time. In an address at the University of Chicago in December 1907 he had come out openly for the general principle: the heads of clinical departments "should devote their main energies and time to their hospital work and to teaching and investigating without the necessity of seeking their livelihood in a busy outside practice and without allowing such practice to become their chief professional occupation." In 1910 he attempted without success to apply this principle in the creation of a clinical department for the great Austrian pediatrician Clemens von Pirquet, the effectual founder of the concept of allergy. Here the matter had rested till Welch by his choice of Mall — and Mall's best friend Halsted — to confer with Abraham Flexner predetermined the character of Flexner's report. By March 1911, when Flexner presented his case to the trustees of the university, Welch was "more radically outspoken" than ever before; any doubts or fears had vanished. In June the trustees, under the guidance of Welch, approved the principle of full-time (with the reversion to the university of all fees from private practice), subject to the consent of the medical faculty.

The bitterest controversy in the history of the medical school then broke loose, with Welch as interested arbiter. Osler in Oxford began to get reports on the proposed reform in April 1911 and lost no time in writing to his correspondents in Baltimore that the whole idea was "Utopian." He resented the implication that the clinical professors had made themselves rich — "I did not take away from B a dollar made in practice" — but beyond this he deplored the effort to shrink the clinical men to the dimensions of a laboratory. "What would the school have been if the clinical men had not been active in the local and national societies. Would whole-time men have the same influence in the profession at large — I doubt it." But Osler did not get really angry until a copy of Flexner's report to Gates reached him in August "full of errors and misconceptions" including as he thought unmerited aspersions on his protégé Howard Kelly. Osler determined to write an open letter of protest to President Ira Remsen and had copies printed for distribution to the interested parties in America. "I fear," he wrote to Remsen, "lest the broad open spirit which has characterized the school should narrow, as teacher and student chased each other down the fascinating road of research, forgetful of those wider interests to which a great hospital must minister."

From this time forward there was no doubt that full-time could be floated, if at all, only at the cost of lasting ill-will and the probable splitting in two of the medical faculty, the "very happy band" who had always pulled together. Osler's determination to take an active part in the controversy would in itself have produced a grave crisis; but to this was added the ironic fact that Barker, who had made the idea of full-time famous, now concluded that he could not give up the lucrative private practice which he had acquired since coming to Baltimore. He would not stand in the way of reform, but he would not embody it or be the symbol of an effortless transition. There would have to be a new professor of medicine. At least one disciple of Mall had grown away from him.

Welch responded to these difficulties by doing nothing at all except to foster informal discussion. The trustees had given their approval in the late spring of 1911, but the final decision was not reached until October 1913, nearly two and a half years later. From January 1913 to June 1914 Welch was acting president of the university, and could have been the permanent president, but even then he scrupulously avoided any pressure on his colleagues. He kept his own counsel, even more than usual; he had decided to relieve the tension by giving to everyone the sense of having infinite expanses of time in which to conduct the debate. In the meantime Osler kept up from Oxford a drumfire of objections and wrote on one occasion in 1912 that full-time would lead to a faculty of Halsteds — "a very good thing for science, but a very bad thing for the profession."

Abraham Flexner and the others in New York fretted under the long delay. "Why," Flexner wrote to Mall in confidence, "doesn't Dr. Welch either shoot or give up the gun?" When Mall on his own initiative showed the letter to Welch as a means of prodding him, Welch though nettled did not budge but went on waiting. Finally, in October 1913, he as president of the university announced to the General Education Board that the Hopkins would initiate full-time; and the board appropriated $1,500,000 for this purpose.

Osler in disgust said publicly that full-time would probably lead to the production of "a set of clinical prigs, the boundary of whose horizon would be the laboratory, and whose only human interest would be research." By consent of Welch the spirit of Mall — and of himself — now reigned through the whole course of instruction.

Welch took no pleasure in his triumph over Osler, and liked to point out that Osler at the end of his life was urging full-time upon his own alma mater, McGill. But in Baltimore itself the men of Osler's temperament went on thinking for many years that a grave mistake had been made. The chief opponent of full-time among those on the faculty in 1913, Howard Kelly — whose own department of gynecology was not affected for the present — chose to remain and showed his good faith by undertaking new researches. "I don't feel," he wrote the next year, "that I dare hold my position and drift along as I have done in the past. Such is the good result of competition and all-time service in the other departments."

If Howard Kelly was too great a man to be resentful or harbor grudges, others were resentful for him, and for Osler and themselves. This was the price that had to be paid for retaining leadership in the reform of medical education. Welch by his forbearance and good temper had reduced the price to a minimum, but he and his name and the name of the Hopkins had come to be a national possession and could not be sacrificed to local considerations, even their own. The image of the ideal Hopkins had to be projected with all possible sharpness even at the cost of inflicting great strains and pressures on the actual structure. From 1913 forward to 1939 the principled objections to full-time for the leading men in clinical departments grew increasingly faint; and all progressive schools gravitated toward full-time.

In 1913 Welch was sixty-three and might have been expected to regard the introduction of full-time as a last contribution to consolidating the position of the medical school and retaining for it the initiative in reform. But he had already begun to be drawn along into still another experiment. In 1908 he had helped to secure for the medical zoologist Charles Wardell Stiles a place on Theodore Roosevelt's Country Life Commission so that Stiles might "do something for the 'poor whites' of the South." A representative of the Rockefeller General Education Board, Wallace Buttrick, attended some of the sessions as an observer and spent most of one night learning from Stiles about the tragedy of hookworm disease in the South. In October 1909, after much investigation, John D. Rockefeller, Jr. convened a group including Stiles, Welch, and Simon Flexner and invited them to make plans for spending up to one million dollars in combating hookworm over a period of five years. The success of the campaign that followed — the first great public health "demonstration" in America — under the prim-looking educator Wickliffe Rose showed the need for similar efforts on a continuing basis and resulted in the creation, under the auspices of the Rockefeller Foundation, of an International Health Commission.

As the plans of this commission grew steadily more ambitious, the total absence in the United States of any provision for training public health workers became intolerable. In December 1913 the Rockefeller Foundation asked the General Education Board to look into the question of personnel for public health work. At the resulting conference, in October 1914, the three dominant figures were Wickliffe Rose, Hermann M. Biggs, now State Commissioner of Health for New York, and Welch. Biggs, overwhelmed by the difficulty of finding public health officers, at first favored a low level of instruction capable of turning out large numbers of men in the shortest possible time. Welch, as president of the Maryland State Board of Health, had almost as much experience as Biggs with the problem of placing scientifically competent men in public health posts. But he took the opposite stand from Biggs, and argued that the only solution to the difficulty of finding public health personnel was a university department of hygiene on the German model — ". . . everybody knows the risk of starting men too soon in technical training without a good knowledge of general principles." Welch had never forgotten his contact thirty years before with the founder of the laboratory tradition in hygiene, Max von Pettenkofer of Munich. He now spoke in Pettenkofer's spirit. When Wickliffe Rose seconded the proposal for a university connection and sketched the outlines of a great central institute of hygiene presiding over a hierarchy of lesser units as "the directive force," Biggs agreed that this would meet the objects that he had in view and more.

The question of where to place the central institute was resolved by commissioning Abraham Flexner to make a survey. For him the only thing that mattered was to have Welch as first director. From this it followed that the university affiliation must be with Johns Hopkins. Welch was becoming more and more dilatory and unable to screw himself to the point of preparing memoranda, so that his proposals for an institute did not reach the General Education Board until May 1915. A year later an initial appropriation of $267,000 for "a school or institute of hygiene and public health" at Johns Hopkins was made by the Rockefeller Foundation. In the interval, former President Eliot of Harvard had done his best to wreck the scheme.

The grant required that Welch withdraw from all other work at the Hopkins and devote his full time to the new institute. In 1917 he therefore resigned as professor of pathology after thirty-three years, in favor of his own student W. G. MacCallum. Welch continued to be a member of the governing body of the medical school, and would come in late to its meetings and march around to his accustomed chair and stand quietly behind it until whoever was sitting in it got up and let him have it. In the planning of the School of Hygiene and Public Health, he had associated with him as assistant director the physiologist Howell, who had also severed his connections with the medical school. Much of the routine work, and other work as well, fell on the younger man.

When the new school opened its doors in October 1918 — with seventeen students, the same number with which the medical school had begun — Welch's contribution to its success had in great part already been made. He had insisted on a generous conception of the nature of instruction in public health, not bacteriology alone, but this together with everything that Pettenkofer had taught at Munich and more; engineering, demography, parasitology, biochemistry. Only Welch had the power to make second-rate instruction in the field unnegotiable. To maintain the standard that he had laid down, he and Howell chose a strong faculty, including most notably the great student of vitamins E. V. McCollum.

Once the school had opened, Welch had no very serious responsibilities other than policy-making and the gradual filling out of the staff. But once a week he gave a lecture on "selected topics in hygiene." Often he talked about the great sanitarians of the past, like Edwin Chadwick, or demographers like John Graunt and William Farr, and portrayed the history of health and disease as a function of broad social developments, like the Industrial Revolution. Yet his role as a teacher was essentially peripheral and the School of Hygiene and Public Health, unlike the medical school, was a structure which he had built but could not really enter into. To this necessity he consented with dignity and candor.

None of this could take from him the distinction of having added a third major unit to the medical institutions of the university, concerned, unlike the hospital and medical school, with the prevention rather than the treatment of disease. In 1922 the Rockefeller Foundation placed its seal of approval upon the new enterprise in Baltimore by granting an endowment of $6,000,000. All over the world, schools of hygiene were created by the Rockefeller Foundation on the Baltimore model — in London, Toronto, and Copenhagen, São Paulo, Zagreb, and Prague,

Tokyo, Ankara, and Sofia; and the directors of many of these institutions went to Johns Hopkins for training. Welch had proved in a second spurt of creativity that vitality and capacity for leadership had not departed from the Hopkins with Osler.

XIII
The Apotheosis of an Influential

On one of his frequent trips to Europe, Welch found himself in Munich at the end of July 1914, with crowds coursing through the streets crying, *"Deutschland über Alles"* and intolerant of anyone who held back. Welch wisely got up on a chair and sang as indicated: Deutschland over everything. "It is all quite thrilling, but a general European war is too horrible to contemplate, and it seems impossible that it will occur."

By the middle of August, Welch was trapped by the impossible war in the neutral pocket of Switzerland and wondering which way to turn in his effort to get back home. He ended by making for England via France and reached New York without incident. His whole impulse, at least at the outset, seems to have been not to take sides but to regard the war as a dreadful fate that had overtaken everybody together: the "horror and disgrace" attached not to the warring parties but to the war itself. His state of mind fell in with the disinterested revulsion from the whole idea of warfare which characterized the first period of Wilson's war diplomacy.

Welch expected Wilson to keep the United States out of the war, and from 1914 to the spring of 1916 his own activities were not much affected by events in Europe. He was then passing through one of his creative periods at the Hopkins, with the founding of the School of Hygiene. Moreover, he spent the last months of 1915 on the other side of the world.

As a counterpart of the economic penetration of China by the Standard Oil Company, the Rockefeller Foundation had taken as one of its first projects the introduction into China of Western medicine and medical instruction. In the summer of 1915 the China Medical Board, a subsidiary of the foundation, sent a commission to the Orient to survey medical education there and to transform the Peking Union Medical College into a school of the first class. The members included Wallace Buttrick, Gates, Simon Flexner, and Welch. Welch had gone on to Hawaii ahead of the others, who picked him up en route to Japan. At the inevitable ceremonial dinners Welch was supplied as a mark of distinction with the youngest possible geisha, who flitted about in a restless way and pressed food upon him, while the other Americans drew older women who were willing to sit still and talk quietly. "Flexner, why do they always give me these children?" Welch would say.

From Japan the party moved on by way of Korea to its real destination, Peking. Here they found a great deal of work to do — to placate the missionaries and assure them that religion would not be the loser by reforms in the medical school; to reconcile the native ancestor worshipers to the practice of dissecting the human body; to persuade the missionaries to make the language of medical instruction English; and to get both groups to agree to coeducation, a subject on which Welch had long since retracted his hostile opinion.

He took as his own special task to give both to the missionaries and to the Chinese themselves a sense of perspective as to where they stood in terms of European history. The date was, he said, about 1600, and the age of Gilbert, Galileo, and Bacon was about to dawn. Those men had stood for "exact observation, experiment and verification of hypotheses by experience" and had thereby displaced in Europe what the Chinese would now also have to give up — "veneration for books, dogma and authority." With this prodding and criticism, Welch combined great enthusiasm for everything in Chinese culture which was no impediment to scientific medicine, particularly art, drama, and food. He tasted all thirty-seven courses of a memorable dinner, from "4000 year eggs" and bird's nest to sharks' fins and Peking duck rolled in pancake, found "nothing really distasteful" and some things delicious, and took great pleasure in the general expectation that he would be "prostrated" by eating more of the wrong things than any other Westerner present. He remained in excellent health.

From China the party returned to Japan at the end of 1915 for sight-seeing. As Welch grew older he made a point of outlasting his younger associates; he now went off alone to see a famous temple and spent the night at a native inn. Here the landlord supplied him with three giggling girls who made a nuisance of themselves at dinner and far from departing at bedtime started to pull off his clothes. After dismissing them with great firmness, he still had misgivings. Flushing the three of them from their hiding place behind a screen, he sent them squealing away. "It is apparent," he wrote in his diary, "that the girls are there for other purposes than as maid-servants."

In 1916 Welch returned from this carefree tourist life to the growing threat of war in the United States. Earlier, he had rejected as president of the National Academy of Sciences a proposal by the astronomer George Ellery Hale to offer the services of American science to the President in the event of war. At the end of April, however, he presided over a meeting of the academy which voted unanimously to inform Wilson "that in the event of a break in diplomatic relations with any country, the Academy desires to place itself at the disposal of the Government for any services within its scope." Wilson agreed to receive a delegation led by Welch and told the academy to go ahead with its plans, but not to say anything in public.

Hale, with Welch's co-operation, began at once to lay plans for a National Research Council, more inclusive than the academy and less weighted toward the side of age. Wilson agreed in July to let the whole matter be brought out into the open. Hale, who deeply resented American neutrality, was now free to go to Europe and confer with the English and French scientists. He and Welch sailed together in August 1916. But even at this late date, when Hale, like Theodore Roosevelt, was breathing fire from every pore, Welch was not primarily concerned with the war. His principal objects in going abroad were to get advice on the School of Hygiene and to find a successor to Howell as professor of physiology. He now regarded the English physiologists as the ablest in the world.

In Oxford he visited with the Oslers, now Sir William and Lady Osler, and saw the "very fine fellow" Revere Osler "about 20, in artillery, soon to go to front." But the "wonderful, mysterious, unforgettable" experience was to see London crouching in the darkness with the intermittent searchlights playing across the sky. On a short excursion to France, where he twice went pretty far up toward the front, he visited the hospitals of Alexis Carrel and Sir Almroth Wright and saw the English troops go singing on their way to the trenches — "many to be 'cannon-fodder.'" Of this whole initiation into wartime life in the twentieth century, he wrote to Hale, "What a wonderfully interesting time we have had."

On his return to the United States he soon had to deal with a grave challenge to the National Research Council. A member of Wilson's Council on National Defense named Hollis Godfrey was trying to organize a committee on science with himself as chairman. If this went through, the National Research Council, the real organ of the productive scientists, might find itself with nothing to do. Hale, in Pasadena, California, could hardly contain himself, but the burden of negotiating with the administration fell on Welch, whom Hale favored with a steady stream of communications, uniformly pessimistic. Working in large part through Daniel Willard, in peacetime the president of the Baltimore and Ohio but now a central figure in the preparedness effort, Welch secured in March 1917 official recognition of the National Research Council as the scientific arm of the Council on National Defense. To the distress of Hale, Welch agreed that Godfrey should be a member of the National Research Council — not that there was anything for him to do, "but we have won out and must secure harmony." Within less than a month the United States was at war with Germany. After this one indispensable service Welch largely withdrew from the affairs of the National Research Council. He was now busy with other things.

His old student from the New York quiz of forty years before, William C. Gorgas — for whom Welch had later interceded with Theodore Roosevelt in the matter of the Panama Canal — was now Surgeon General. Immediately after the declaration of war Welch offered his services in any capacity that Gorgas chose. Visitors to the Surgeon General's office in the spring of 1917 were surprised to find Welch encamped in Gorgas's own private room, answering the telephone and handling the mail. Harvey Cushing had some difficulty in keeping his attention on an interview with Gorgas in the — oblivious — presence of Welch. There was certainly an element of humor in Welch's falling-to to clear up someone else's correspondence.

This was a passing episode and by midsummer of 1917 he was ready for other work. In July he received a major's commission in the Medical Section of the Officers' Reserve Corps and began the first of many visits of inspection to military camps throughout the country. When he set out on these tours, which took him as far west as Texas and New Mexico, he was already a man of sixty-seven, but tireless and proud of his ability to keep going after all of his younger associates were reduced to exhaustion. As a rule he went only where there was trouble — measles, pneumonia, or meningitis. He would visit the sick, join in autopsies on the dead, feel the blankets and clothing, look under and over and behind, taste the food, kick up some dust to see what danger there was of respiratory ailments when the wind came whipping through the camp, look at the women round about as possible carriers of venereal disease, count the test tubes in the laboratory, and above all put some spirit, and occasionally a little fear, into the medical men and even the line officers. Then he would send off to Washington a detailed report of what was wrong, what might go wrong in the future, and what ought to be done.

By fall he decided, contrary to his previous opinion, that he needed the prestige of a uniform. He was therefore called to active service in November and rose to colonel by July 1918 — with his fine handsome head with the white mustache and goatee that any commander of troops might have envied, but also a great unmilitary paunch that seemed gently to inflate itself from year to year, and a loose waggle of the fingers as a kind of warrant that an unrepentant civilian was lurking beneath the surface and declined to master the art of saluting.

In the fall of 1918 just as he had persuaded himself that things were well in hand and no longer called for his services, he and everyone else received a bad shock with the outbreak of influenza in the most virulent form in modern times — "some new kind of infection or plague" as Welch called it when the first reports began to come in and seemed to resemble nothing of which anyone had ever heard. After this final crisis, for which Welch had no solution, he secured his release from active service on the last day of December 1918.

Welch's other contribution to the winning of the war had been made almost thirty years before. The most notable of his discoveries in bacteriology had been that of the Welch bacillus which killed people by flooding their systems with gas. Gas gangrene had not been very common in peacetime, but now proved a serious threat to troops on the Western front. At this point a young investigator then in uniform, C. G. Bull, came forward with an antitoxin for the Welch bacillus, and confronted Welch, Gorgas, and the Secretary of War Newton D. Baker with the problem of whether or not to publish a discovery from which the enemy would benefit equally with the Allies. They agreed at once, in Welch's words, that "We should not consider for a moment holding back such a life-saving discovery on the ground that the enemy could also make use of it."

At the close of the war Welch shared in the same apocalyptic vision as Woodrow Wilson that the world could be made radically safe — safe for democracy, safe from disease — safe. Speaking in 1919 Welch went down the list of old enemies of mankind which could now be banished by known methods: typhoid, "once the bane of armies," but now "entirely negligible"; tetanus, "completely controlled"; malaria, "hardly to be bothered with at all"; venereal disease, "reduced to a point never before realized." Among the workers in the field of public health this feeling of euphoria was general; and the year 1919 saw not only Wilson's effort to launch the League of Nations from Paris but another effort, also under American auspices, to put together at Cannes an international Red Cross of enormous power and scope in the sphere of hygiene and preventive medicine.

To this conference Welch and Hermann M. Biggs went as representatives of the American Red Cross. Welch served as presiding officer at most of the sessions. Biggs and some of the other Americans present seemed to think in terms of an international organization acting directly upon the peoples of the world. But Welch, though confident that wonders could be worked, retained his sense of political realities and did his best to keep before the

APOTHEOSIS OF AN INFLUENTIAL 193

delegates the fact that the Red Cross was organized into national units and lacked compulsive powers. The resolutions adopted at Cannes, in which he largely concurred, called for a breath-taking complex of reforms and innovations ranging from the construction of adequate housing for workingmen, through universal instruction in hygiene, to the annihilation of typhus and tuberculosis. The whole program was the high-water mark of the socialism of hygiene as an international enterprise, of a spaciousness that has never even been approached. As it turned out, the League of Red Cross Societies which resulted came to share many of these proposed functions, in so far as they were exercised at all, with the Health Section of the League of Nations and the International Health Board of the Rockefeller Foundation.

On this visit to France in the spring of 1919 Welch lapsed for the first time into calling the Germans "Huns" as he drove through the remains of "the very hell of war" around Verdun. By the time of his next visit to Europe, at the height of the German inflation in 1923, the war hatreds had receded into the past and he was greatly moved by the plight of the investigators on whom he had tried to model his own career — the younger Wilhelm His now dependent for experimental animals on some students from Japan, the bacteriologist Flügge, with whom he himself had studied, apologizing for having a cake in the midst of general want. Welch sent Flügge a check for $50 "with a friendly letter." Welch, who had borne the tradition of scientific medicine from Germany to America forty years before, had now outlived the golden age of the biological sciences in Germany.

He had also begun to outlive his colleagues at Johns

Hopkins. Mall died first, in 1917; Osler, heartbroken at the death of his only son in the war, followed in 1919; and Halsted in 1922. (Howard Kelly lived on till 1943 but withdrew from the Hospital in 1919.) Welch tried in turn to define the contribution of each man: Mall, who had stood for productivity in research; Osler, who must not be thought of primarily as a propagandist for public health — as Harvey Cushing unwisely ventured to suggest — but as the man who had given medical students entry into the wards; Halsted, whom he confessed to admiring "above all my colleagues," a scientific surgeon who shared in the spirit of John Hunter and Claude Bernard. But Welch's principal business in the 1920's was not to strike the elegiac note for departed colleagues or to muse over the past but to go on strengthening the Hopkins as no one else could. In 1924 and 1925 he thus took the lead (with assistance from the General Education Board) in bringing Dr. William H. Wilmer to Baltimore to establish a full-time clinic in ophthalmology and succeeded in raising $600,000 for this purpose in the course of a single morning of interviews in which he blandly took for granted that the philanthropists whom he approached would wish to engage in friendly competition with their checkbooks.

The real challenge of the twenties, however, was to open up a third successive field of study at the Hopkins. When the hospital and medical school were still in the planning stage John Shaw Billings had advocated instruction in the history of medicine. Though no chair in the field had been set up at the Hopkins, Osler had brought into being in 1889 the Johns Hopkins Hospital Historical Club, of which Welch served as first president. With the hearty co-operation of Howard Kelly, they had made this club an important element in the life of the medical institutions. Over the years Welch spoke before the club on themes ranging from Hippocrates, Galen, and the School of Salerno through the history of animal experimentation, to William Harvey, Albrecht von Haller, and Edward Jenner. Some of the best of Osler's historical and biographical essays were also read before the same audience; and the collection of these entitled *An Alabama Student,* published at Oxford in 1908, was dedicated to Welch, "whose unselfish devotion to science illustrates the spirit that in every age has made medicine of service to humanity."

Like Osler, Welch often spoke on historical themes outside Baltimore, most notably perhaps at Albany in 1906 on "Some of the Conditions Which Have Influenced the Development of American Medicine." Unlike Osler, Welch seldom made any systematic use of primary sources, printed or manuscript, and none of his historical papers compares in freshness or scholarship with Osler's "An Alabama Student" or "The Influence of Louis on American Medicine." But at least once, at Philadelphia in 1895, Welch touched in a glancing way on one of the great neglected themes in the history of the nineteenth century, "The Evolution of Modern Scientific Laboratories." Welch had no delusions about his own competence as a historian, but he never lost sight of the desirability of having medical history taught at the Hopkins by the right kind of man.

At the beginning of the 1920's this alone, of all the things that he had envisioned for the university, still remained to be done. For the first time he began to talk of retiring — in 1925, say, when he reached his seventy-fifth birthday. But hardly anyone prominent in American medicine had any recollection of a time when Welch was not active at the center of things; and his friends agreed that he, who seemed to be eternal, would have to be kept in harness by some means. For this purpose they would have to find some new temptation to usefulness, and suddenly, in the spring of 1925, everyone was talking at once of the obvious solution. Welch's colleagues at Johns Hopkins, the pathologist MacCallum and the pediatrician John Howland, wrote to Abraham Flexner in New York; and Flexner, on Welch's invitation, set out once more for Baltimore.

Welch now announced to his visitor that his mind was made up to retire in the immediate future. To his utter astonishment he heard, in place of protestations and regrets, the terse reply that this was undoubtedly a very wise decision. All of the old man's sensitivities were aroused in an instant and he flung out the question with which he had now just begun to live: "Do you think I am losing ground?" "No, but I have another job for you." The conversation was now taking the line for which Welch had prepared himself. "I don't want another job. I want to loaf." But, Flexner went on, he would want this job: "the creation in America of a professorship of the history of medicine." And, he concluded, Welch could do the job easily, and no one else could do it at all.

Welch's friends had chosen their point of attack with great skill. As the chief Influential of American medicine he had sought for more than a generation to render medical instruction thoroughly scientific. In this cause he had recently carried through the full-time reform at Johns Hopkins over the opposition of Osler. But he was always prepared to trim against himself, and, after going one way, to go the other. By reason of his own successes the time had now come to fight for humanism in the medical schools. As he said in 1930, the more medicine became an applied science "the greater the need of the cultivation of the humanistic side of medicine." The history of medicine had more than a "mere dormant, cultural aspect." Of two great men with whom he had collaborated, he pointed out that Osler and Sir Clifford Allbutt were "better physicians, better teachers, and had far greater influence in the profession and in the community by virtue of these literary and cultural interests which I would like to call 'medical humanism.' "

Welch and Osler had once had to trim their personalities to the core, to define the meaning of full-time and display the issues involved. Now Welch in his old age was reunited with Osler in pursuit of fullness of being; and the inner Welch like the outer became more and more ample and inclusive. The accommodation with the spirit of Osler was perfect in the end.

When, therefore, Welch's friends told him in 1925 that there ought to be a chair of the history of medicine at Johns Hopkins, he agreed at once with great enthusiasm. "My dream had been a central library for the hospital, medical school and School of Hygiene, and in connection with this an endowed chair of the history of medicine" — "not merely a cultural centre, important as that is, but a real adjuvant of the development of scientific medicine." Welch's own candidate for the chair was not himself, but the author of the standard history of medicine in English, Fielding H. Garrison. "For me to take such a chair at my age would merely emphasize the spirit of dilettantism in which the subject is regarded and pursued generally in this country." But the General Education Board, from which the money would have to come, made clear that a grant would only be made if Welch himself took the chair. In May 1925 he gave in. Early in 1926 the board made a grant of $200,000 for a professorship of the history of medicine and the building of a medical library to be named after Welch.

Welch had stood at Johns Hopkins and elsewhere for the filling of academic chairs in medicine by men with the most rigorous possible training. He ended his career by becoming the only professor in the medical faculty without such training. For a man of his temperament and incapacity for self-deception this radically false position was often a torment — to be, as he wrote to the Harvard historian of science George Sarton in 1930, "only an interloper" in the field. His last service to Johns Hopkins was to purchase for it a medical library and the endowment of a new chair at the sacrifice of ideals that he had kept fresh and vulnerable through a long life. But even in yielding on the matter of scholarly competence, he remained incorruptible and always kept before him the two objects of laying a proper foundation for rigorous work and quickly finding a successor more fit than himself to build upon it.

In spite of these reservations, Welch took great pleasure in the task of shopping for books for the new library. From May 1927 to September 1928 he wandered over Europe for the last time, with many pauses for relaxation, and made the circuit of the great continental and British booksellers. The philosophy behind his purchases was if not undiscriminating extremely generous, and almost any book about history might qualify. In the course of this long *Wanderjahr* he came to depend heavily on the bibliophile Arnold Klebs of Nyon, Switzerland, the son of a pioneer bacteriologist whom he had known fifty years before. But even this long pleasure-and-business excursion soon took on a nightmare aspect as Welch duplicated his own purchases and juggled despairingly with catalogues and accounts rendered (all on different systems) and spent many times over the amount originally appropriated for the purpose.

If Welch was not the ideal man to stock a great library, he had always known how to find the best man in any field and become his student. He therefore went to the most distinguished of all medical historians, Karl Sudhoff, of the Institute of the History of Medicine at Leipzig, for advice. Welch had already determined that a single professor was not enough, and that a group of scholars would have to be organized into an institute on Sudhoff's pattern. His visit to Leipzig merely confirmed this view. Sudhoff told him that the first of the younger medical historians was Henry Sigerist, "perhaps as more brilliant and stirring and full of ideas on organization than as a solid, steady, thorough investigator." The next ranking man, Paul Diepgen, Sudhoff described as more thorough, sound, and laborious than Sigerist.

Back in Baltimore Welch presided over the opening of the William H. Welch Library in October 1929. In May 1930 the General Education Board made a final appropriation of $250,000 to endow a true institute as distinguished from a single professorship, with additional funds to finance the work of the first five years. Every purpose for which Welch had ever sought money from a foundation had now been fulfilled.

In April 1930 Welch reached his eightieth birthday, and his friends contrived against all expectation to make the occasion climactic for a man whose more important birthdays had been celebrated in a mounting crescendo since 1910. President Hoover agreed to speak in Welch's honor, over an international hookup, and celebrations were held in the leading medical centers of the United States, in London, Paris, Geneva, Tokyo, Peking — and Norfolk, Connecticut. The President struck the inevitable note and called Welch "our greatest statesman in the field of public health." Welch said in reply that he would be "overpowered with a sense of unreality depriving me of utterance" if he thought that this was merely a personal tribute; but he would take it instead as a tribute through him to "an army of teachers, investigators, pupils, associates, and colleagues" who had raised scientific medicine and public health to an "eminent" position in the eyes of their fellow men. If he, for his part, had "handed on any intellectual heritage to pupils, assistants, and associates," he and they were in the debt of "my own masters." "America is now paying the debt which she has owed so long to the Old World by her own active and fruitful participation in scientific discovery and the advancement of the science and art of medicine and sanitation." But, he concluded, "much more remains to be done than has been accomplished," and no one ought to be complacent or self-satisfied.

In the summer of 1930 Welch spent three months at the Huntington Library in San Marino, California, ostensibly making a survey of their resources in the history of medicine and science, but actually browsing to his heart's content. He also went to hear Aimee Semple MacPherson and found her appeal "fundamentally sexual," had tea with Mary Pickford and Douglas Fairbanks, and appeared with them "in the talkies" for a newsreel.

On his return to the East, he had still to cope with the one remaining problem of his life, the choice of an appropriate successor as professor of the history of medicine and head of the institute. Charles Singer, the leading British historian of biology and medicine, refused an invitation secured for him by Welch over much opposition; and the next choice, Harvey Cushing, though he gave no definitive response, probably had no intention of accepting in the end. Here the matter stood in the fall of 1931 when Henry Sigerist came to America and made a powerful impression wherever he spoke. Welch had previously referred to Sigerist's political leanings as one possible danger attaching to his appointment; but the mention of this point seems to have been merely an expedient for procuring the choice of Singer. Welch himself had taken part in a protest meeting for Sacco and Vanzetti; and when President Gilman's daughter was nominated for governor of Maryland by the Socialists in 1930, he wrote to say that though not a Socialist he found much in the program of her party to sympathize with. The unthinking prejudice against Socialism in America, he said, would be "quite incomprehensible" in western Europe. Sigerist's politics were therefore no real barrier in Welch's eyes. In May 1932 Sigerist, after having his doubts resolved by the turn of events in Germany, agreed to come to Baltimore as Welch's successor.

Once again Welch had filled a chair at Johns Hopkins with the strongest possible man; and now at eighty-two he secured his final release from active service. After a few months of comparative leisure — and pulling for Hoover against Franklin Roosevelt because "I did so much resent Roosevelt's stab at the League of Nations" — he entered the Johns Hopkins Hospital with cancer in February 1933 and never left. As the weight fell away from him, he remained uncomplaining and alert and kept his doctors enthralled with recollections of the past. He never asked any questions about his condition and made no gestures toward religion. Biologists, he said, were more skeptical than physicists, and few biologists had any conception of life after death.

When he died on April 30, 1934, he had just turned eighty-four. He had lived from the world of *Middlemarch* into the world of *Arrowsmith:* from the world in which the only betrayal of scientific medicine was to go in pursuit of money into the world of foundations, research institutes, and propaganda assaults on disease. He had made for himself and others many opportunities for lapsing from research into administration, policy-making, and the marshaling of opinion. But from this amplification of the moral dilemmas of the man of scientific medicine he had saved himself whole by self-knowledge and unfailing humility in the presence of research.

An Afterword, 1987

As with any biography published over thirty years ago, anyone who reads or, conceivably, rereads this life of William H. Welch is entitled to ask three main questions. What light has subsequent research thrown upon Welch and his immediate collaborators? What further developments have altered the general context in which he operated? How far have his principal achievements survived and, a more searching test, how far have they maintained their pertinence from our present perspective? Given the centrality of Welch's position, answering these questions entails pondering what has become of American medicine since this book was written.

Largely no doubt because of the prior existence of a spacious and admirable life of Welch by Simon Flexner and James T. Flexner (*William Henry Welch and the Heroic Age of American Medicine*: New York, 1941), no further biographies of Welch have been published other than the present book. Harvey Cushing's vast and delightful biography of Sir William Osler (Oxford, 1925) has forestalled any major reinterpretations of him. His nephew, Dr. W. W. Francis, in a letter to the author indignantly denied that Osler had migrated to Oxford to receive a knighthood, or ever craved that distinction, which Howard Kelly (as reported in this book) had once told a colleague was Osler's great ambition in life. We still lack a large-scale biography of the great surgeon William Stewart Halsted; but on a point of which much was made in the present book, we now have reason to suppose that he never completely broke his addiction to cocaine but had numerous lapses. This only makes his surgical record at Johns Hopkins all the more remarkable. Presumably it also means that Welch had to go on periodically renewing his faith in Halsted over the whole of their time together. A short popular life of the fourth great figure from the heroic days at Johns Hopkins, Howard Kelly, did appear—Audrey W. Davis's *Dr. Kelly of Hopkins: Surgeon, Scientist, Christian* (Baltimore, 1959)—with the indicated emphasis upon the pervasiveness of Christianity in Kelly's life. The generosity of spirit with which he accepted the decision to move toward "full-time" appointments for clinical professors is shown by Davis to have been characteristic of the man. Toward evil or corruption, however, he was unrelenting.

The liveliest evocations of an entire set of people with whom Welch significantly interacted are given by John Ettling in his book on the campaign against hookworm disease, *The Germ of Laziness: Rockefeller Philanthropy and Public Health in the New South* (Cambridge, Massachusetts, 1981). This is a work of much broader scope than the title might indicate, amounting to a group portrait of the Rockefellers, father and son, and their main philanthropic counsellors. Welch himself, as the principal adviser to them in creating the Rockefeller Institute, came in close contact (then and later) with the fabulous Frederick T. Gates, a Baptist clergyman who had gone hat in hand for a benefaction from the elder Rockefeller only to be sized up as a good man to cope with the innumerable other suppliants for a piece of Rockefeller's fortune. Gates ended by becoming the main *business* adviser to Rockefeller as well.

As set forth in the present book, Gates in later years made an ultimately famous speech to a group of scientists at the Rockefeller Institute, in which he said, to some initial merriment from the audience, that medical research would be promulgating "new moral laws and new social laws, new definitions of what is right and wrong in our relations with each other." The piquancy of these remarks has always been seen as lying in the fact that a devout Baptist clergyman could have been brought to locate the wellsprings of future morality in science. But Ettling, drawing upon Gates's belatedly published autobiography, *Chapters in My Life* (New York, 1977), has now shown that Gates had already abandoned Baptist fundamentalism before signing on with Rockefeller. Against a vaguely theistic backdrop, Gates had become essentially a secular reformer early in his career and in no need of being persuaded that, building upon the foundation laid by a merely human Jesus, people would have to make and remake their own morals on a continually evolving basis. Gates did not have to learn from others to put science above religion or rather to devolve upon science what he regarded as the main function of traditional religion, to embody our desire and capacity to improve the human lot. The key figure in the Rockefeller philanthropies had converted to the primacy of science long before Welch and other medical leaders first encountered him.

On Johns Hopkins as Welch's native environment, Dean

Alan M. Chesney published before his death two further volumes of his self-styled "chronicle," *The Johns Hopkins Hospital and the Johns Hopkins University School of Medicine* (Baltimore, 1958, 1963), covering between them the period from 1893 to 1914, precisely when Welch was in his prime. Though calculatedly uninterpretative, these volumes contain many previously unpublished documents of great interest, including letters and confidential memoranda about the abortive efforts to recruit the brilliant Austrian pediatrician Clemens von Pirquet, the totally unanticipated windfall of Henry Phipps's offer to create a psychiatric clinic and Adolf Meyer's implementation of this, and the bitterly contested decision to move toward full-time for clinical professors.

Chesney inevitably conjoined the Johns Hopkins Hospital and the Johns Hopkins Medical School as equal components of a unitary whole, as stipulated by the founder himself. Nobody has ever failed to see that this was an essential condition for what was accomplished in Baltimore. But neither the present book nor any other had adequately grasped the true distinctiveness of the situation till Kenneth M. Ludmerer's *Learning to Heal: The Development of American Medical Education* (New York, 1985). He there showed that the greatest single impediment to improving medical education, once this had become a widely recognized necessity, was the almost insuperable difficulty of persuading the old established hospitals, touchily proud of their independence and skittish about turning medical students loose upon their patients, to become *teaching* hospitals closely affiliated with new or reformed medical schools. The paradox became that cities with some of the best existing hospitals and some of the more respectable of the older medical schools, had the greatest difficulty in forging an alliance between them.

Ludmerer tells the cautionary tale of Roosevelt Hospital, the most flourishing and probably the most progressive hospital in New York City around 1900 but mulishly resisting repeated overtures from the College of Physicians and Surgeons of Columbia University to become its teaching affiliate. P&S finally took no for an answer and turned instead to Presbyterian Hospital. Roosevelt speedily declined to a stodgily respectable hospital of the second rank while Presbyterian forged ahead. In Boston, the great Massachusetts General Hospital just barely saved itself from inevitable decline by affiliating with the Harvard Medical School as late as 1912, and then only because the newly founded Brigham Hospital had been a Harvard teaching hospital from the start and the sudden competition for staff and prestige had driven MGH grudgingly into Harvard's arms. Welch and his colleagues at Johns Hopkins had had almost a generation of lead time over Harvard and Columbia because the existing hospitals in New York and Boston were too important to ignore and too foolish to welcome the association that would save them. The unique stature of the Johns Hopkins Medical School in its formative period was a function not only of the founder's wisdom and the vision and distinction of Welch and his colleagues but also of the fact that New York and Boston were severely hobbled by the hospital situation.

One of the closest observers of the experiment in Baltimore and the principal trumpeter of its virtues was the layman Abraham Flexner, successively employed by the Carnegie and Rockefeller philanthropies. Great emphasis is laid in this book upon Flexner's famous report for the

Carnegie Foundation for the Advancement of Teaching, *Medical Education in the United States and Canada* (New York, 1910), candidly premised on the necessity for all other medical schools to resemble Johns Hopkins as fast as possible or to go out of business. Probably no single issue about the history of medical reform in America has been as actively canvassed in recent years as the exact significance and impact of the Flexner Report. Among the main contributors to the debate have been Daniel M. Fox ("Abraham Flexner's Unpublished Report: Foundations and Medical Education, 1909–1928," *Bulletin of the History of Medicine*, 54 (1980), 475–496) and Kenneth M. Ludmerer. Since Flexner saw himself as propagating the gospel according to Welch, the issue is correspondingly important for Welch's own impact. The general verdict seems to be that the Flexner Report has been overrated. The evidence is clear that proprietary, i.e., strictly commercial, schools were on the wane and rapidly closing down in the years immediately *before* the Report. On the positive side of these developments, no knowledgeable person has ever suggested that Flexner initiated the efforts at improving medical education in the better though highly imperfect schools. He was eloquently articulating, with cautionary examples to the contrary, an ideal that was already on the way to prevailing if he had never published a word on the subject. The independently potent example of Johns Hopkins had to precede his own efforts, as he would have been the first to insist. Nevertheless, Flexner strengthened the hand of those who were fighting to upgrade their own medical schools and badly in need of reenforcement from an aroused public opinion. And if the scandalously bad schools were already falling by the wayside, he undoubtedly fostered mass suicide among the survivors. The effort to cut Flexner and his Report down to size has gone too far. He was a great man who did a great work.

One of the main ingredients in Flexner's, and Welch's, prescription for medical schools was laboratories in physiology and experimental pathology. This inevitably elicited an outcry from antivivisectionists and efforts by them to obtain severe legislative restraints upon animal experimentation. This became one of Welch's main concerns from the 1890s forward. In the absence of any serious historical literature on this topic, the account of antivivisectionism in this book was necessarily impressionistic. We now have two overlapping though differently focussed scholarly works on the rise of antivivisection, its leaders and their motivations, and the degree of success that they attained—Richard D. French, *Antivivisection and Medical Science in Victorian Society* (Princeton, 1975) and James Turner, *Reckoning with the Beast: Animals, Pain, and Humanity in the Victorian Mind* (Baltimore, 1980). The principal light that these books cast upon Welch's situation is the late emergence and overwhelmingly derivative character of the antivivisectionist impulse in America, with virtually all the arguments lifted bodily from English writers and the horrible examples drawn from alleged abuses in Europe, and hoary abuses at that, dating from far back. Even its worst enemies could never come up with much evidence that animal experimentation was being sadistically pursued by Welch's generation in America. This did not of course moderate the antivivisectionists' indignation.

With the possible exception of Frederick T. Gates's intellectual and spiritual pilgrimage, few of the things that historians have laboriously uncovered about the people and events of his own lifetime would have come as a surprise to Welch, with his incomparable ringside seat for everything that was going on in medicine. But what would he have made of developments in the fifty years since he died? Or, differently put, what can we perceive to have been the salient respects in which the medical world as he knew it has been altered out of all recognition?

One of the most poignant changes from his own point of view would have been the apparently irrevocable decline of German science, the lodestar of his own career. He himself had seen the ravages wrought upon it by the First World War. But the 1920s and for that matter the very early 1930s had appeared to put Germany back in the saddle scientifically, though (as he fully appreciated) more on the side of the physical sciences than the biological or medical. In the fifty-two years since Welch's death, only five Germans living and working in Germany have received Nobel Prizes for physiology or medicine, and some of the researches in question dated from an earlier period. By this admittedly crude measure, the supremacy of American science has become overwhelming, though in proportion to a much smaller population scientists in Britain have kept pace with the Americans in becoming Nobelists. Many leading scientists in both countries in the last fifty years were, of course, German or Austrian refugees; but the United States and Britain had become, with Hitler's assistance, indubitably the best environments for doing science. In a way, American supremacy in science was precisely the consummation of Welch's youthful desires, but he would almost certainly have been saddened to see Germany virtually out of the running.

AN AFTERWORD

The vigor of American medical research at the end of the twentieth century would have been gratifying to Welch, but he would probably have been troubled, if not dismayed, by some of the terms on which this had been achieved. On one of the main issues, he might well have been assailed by misgivings about his own role in pointing the way. The nub of the great confrontation over full-time between himself and Osler had been whether an irreparable rift was being opened between the whole of the medical professoriate and the body of ordinary practitioners, as even the clinical professors retreated into a monastic seclusion from the rest of the profession. Full-time never became as universal or as air-tight as Osler feared, and there were many other factors fostering resentment toward medical researchers by the foot soldiers of the profession who bore the heat of battle. But there can be no doubt that Welch was the key figure in creating an aloof cadre of elite researchers serving the actual patient only at many removes. The whole issue flared up at the end of the 1960s when many medical students thought that the best among them were being pointed by their professors toward careers in research when the urgent need was for hands-on practice at the bedside. That was a special moment in history; but the tension between research and practice, researchers and practitioners, has become perennial. Welch himself transcended it by serving as president of the American Medical Association in 1910, but at the end of the twentieth century it is hardly conceivable that the "working" physicians of America would choose an academic investigator to speak for them. That would almost be a contradiction in terms, and Welch, despite his capacity for straddling the gap, was one of those who created it.

Forewarned by the bitterness of the "full-time" controversy, Welch must have been ruefully resigned to some such division in the medical ranks. He also had ample warning that basic research was not going to be confined to the universities, as he would undoubtedly have preferred. Unless he had been prepared to forfeit his preeminence in American medicine, he had been obliged to take the lead in creating in the Rockefeller Institute a richly endowed rival to Johns Hopkins and other medical schools. He had also been chairman of the executive board of the Carnegie Institution of Washington, with its policy of endowing essentially independent research establishments that did not have to be associated with universities, though some in effect were.

What nothing in his experience would have prepared Welch for was the gigantic role that the federal government was destined to play, directly and indirectly, in all of the sciences, but particularly in medicine. He had never been a doctrinaire opponent of a strong national government intervening to promote the general welfare. His time in Germany had inoculated him against laissez-faire, and he had swung his weight behind the creation of the United States Public Health Service in 1902. As president of the National Academy of Sciences, he had conscripted American science for the First World War. But that had been an emergency, science had promptly mustered out after the war, and the public health service remained in Welch's eyes a unique function that only the government could perform.

On the issue that lay nearest to his own heart, funding for scientific research in universities, when Welch died in 1934 they and university hospitals were almost totally independent of the federal government. All university research, including scientific, was being financed by the institution itself or out of the investigator's own pocket, eked out by foundation grants of the sort that Welch had helped to initiate early in the century. Less than twenty years after his death, scientific budgets in the universities had been vastly swollen by a quantum jump in the size and cost of equipment, and the federal government had grown accustomed (in wartime) to unprecedented expenditures on science. The two factors imploded to create a situation in which the federal government was the only conceivable source of enough money to keep university science going, and newly amenable to playing this role. After 1950, virtually the whole scientific enterprise in American universities, public and private alike, would simply have closed down without perpetual infusions of federal funds. The Rubicon had been crossed with a vengeance and there could be no turning back.

The universities were permanently tied by a golden shackle to a generally enlightened federal government. There were bound to be fluctuations in Washington's generosity, but the dependence would always be there and all the more when the purse strings were being tightened. In the larger sense, scientific research in America had been politicized, pitched into the political arena once and for all. So long as this was confined to global allocations in the federal budget, eventually fined down to adjudication upon grant proposals by peer reviews, the universities had nothing to fear except the inherent volatility of the whole process.

From the point of view of a university medical scientist like Welch, the truly ominous development was the transformation of the Hygiene Laboratory of the United States Public Health Service into a National Institute of Health as early as 1930, followed by a National Cancer Institute in 1937. After the Second World War, new National Institutes of Health proliferated. These were independent centers of basic research rivalling and outrivalling the greatest medical schools and irresistibly appealing to members of Congress even when the administration of the day was trying to put the brakes on. More Nobelists have been based upon the National Institutes of Health than upon the Johns Hopkins Medical School. In one sense, it does not matter where good medical research is coming from; but from the perspective of medical educators, it is possible to feel that the finite supply of first-rate investigators is being spread increasingly thin and diverted from medical faculties, and the accompanying contact with medical students, by the almost reflex propensity of Congress to go on multiplying National Institutes of Health every time a health problem attracts general attention. One thing is certain: a man of Welch's generation would have been startled by this development.

Welch would have been interested in where medical research was being done, but chiefly he would have been interested in medical progress and the state of public health. Here he would have been confronted by the consummation of his fondest dreams, yet culminating in a malaise that he could never even have imagined. He himself had seen pernicious anemia cured by the researches of one of his own students, and diabetes mellitus brought under control by insulin. But that was merely the beginning. He died on the eve of the introduction of sulfa drugs and, more significantly, just before Howard Florey touched Alexander Fleming's discovery of penicillin into therapeutic usefulness. The antibiotic revolution that followed, complemented by other drugs and new vaccines against viral diseases, understandably led to euphoria about the boons of scientific medicine. Tuberculosis substantially disappeared from advanced societies, polio was licked and smallpox on the verge of worldwide extinction. By 1962, the great immunologist Sir Macfarlane Burnet was proclaiming "the virtual elimination of infectious disease as a significant factor in social life—something that has passed into history." That was a grave exaggeration. Nature still had nasty tricks in store requiring all the ingenuity of medical science to circumvent. Yet even in the face of the AIDS epidemic, the optimism expressed by Burnet has persisted in the chastened form of supposing that when new infectious diseases arise, cures and preventives can surely be found.

The malaise about modern medicine that can never be dispelled turns precisely upon the fact that, in the measure that infectious diseases are successfully dealt with, more and more people will survive into old age to become the natural prey of degenerative diseases, particularly cancer, heart disease, and diabetes. Progress is being made in coping with these also, but in a statistically aging population, putting these advances at the patients' disposal as they go from one barely surmounted crisis to the next is threatening to swamp the health facilities and the health budget of countries committed to making medical services freely available to old people.

Medicare made the United States such a country. This inexorably, though belatedly, forced the federal government to rein in medical and hospital costs; and comparable pressures have arisen in the field of privately financed health plans for younger people. This is all part of a much larger story, admirably told by Paul Starr in *The Social Transformation of American Medicine* (New York, 1982), entailing the ever-increasing emphasis upon medical care as a blatantly economic transaction, stripped of any genial disguises and distastefully symbolized for many people by the rise of commercial hospital companies. The economic aspects of medicine were always there, and always vital, but now they are threatening to become the palpably dominant consideration in an enterprise that people would rather not think of in such terms. They do not like to think of doctors under the thumb of accountants. Welch, as dean of a medical school and the beneficiary on its behalf of big Rockefeller gifts, had well understood that scientific medicine was expensive even before 1914, but perhaps he too would find the present obsession with costs disquieting, if inevitable. Yet he would have to concede that this was merely the dark side of the medical triumphs that he had tried to pave the way for. Medical progress is in danger of outstripping the means of putting it into practice. More profoundly, it is bumping up against the ultimate reality that degenerative ailments can never be permanently fended off in a world that needs to be rid of us at some point.

Apart from these existential and virtually cosmic issues, Welch would be intensely curious about the fortunes of his own beloved Johns Hopkins. As even he must have known, by the time of his death the medical school had entered a period of relative decline, aggravated by the Great Depression and the Second World War. After the war, the medical faculty had to be rebuilt almost from the ground up. Perhaps the key figure in the recovery of Johns Hopkins was the surgeon Alfred Blalock, best known to the general public for his collaboration with Helen Taussig in saving "blue" babies. On the last of his endeavors at Johns Hopkins, Welch would probably have been disappointed by the subsequent development of the history of medicine as a field of research and teaching. His own Institute of the History of Medicine has had a succession of distinguished directors, and other medical schools, notably Yale, have vigorous programs in this field; but perhaps it is fair to say that none of these efforts has exerted the major humanizing influence upon medical students that he had hoped for. Everything else in medical school seems to be more urgent.

Welch was a modest man, but if at the end of his life he had been magically transported to the present, he could hardly have helped wondering who had been the Welches of the intervening fifty years, the Influentials who had knitted the American scientific community together and represented it to society at large. He would have had no difficulty in identifying the physical scientists James B. Conant and Vannevar Bush as the towering Influentials of the Second World War, the organizers of science for victory, and after the war the chief propagandists for the necessity of supporting basic science out of federal funds in peacetime. In the medical sciences broadly conceived, Welch would instantly have recognized that his own nearest equivalent in the period from 1950 to 1970 had been the biophysicist Detlev Bronk, president of the Johns Hopkins University, Rockefeller University (formerly Rockefeller Institute), and the National Academy of Sciences. But in sharp contrast to Welch, who had become a representative figure in American culture at large and the embodiment of scientific medicine for lay people, Bronk remained virtually unknown to the general public though wielding immense authority among the scientists themselves.

Paradoxically, the creation (and revival after a lapse) of

the post of Science Adviser to the President of the United States has not had the effect of propelling this person to national celebrity; even in the scientific community itself, the only truly commanding figure to have held the job has been the chemist George Kistiakowsky. Kistiakowsky did simultaneously enjoy the high esteem of President Eisenhower and the scientists themselves. But this already diminished scope for a scientific Influential has become increasingly difficult to sustain even if Presidents were prepared to look for people with the requisite professional standing. As many questions of scientific concern have become profoundly politicized from their bearing upon nuclear disarmament and foreign policy, there may well be a basic complementarity at work by which the President's Science Adviser can scarcely hope to retain the confidence of the scientific community. Advisers have to preserve their credibility with the President, and they become correspondingly suspect as creatures of the President when addressing other scientists. Alternatively, one of the easiest ways to attract a following among one's fellow scientists has become to assume a fiercely adversarial posture toward the current administration, whichever that may be. Yet an Influential in Welch's mode owed part of his efficacy to having easy access to Presidents who trusted his good will toward them and his abstention from politics. Influentials within the confines of particular fields of specialization will always exist. Science would not work without them. But after Conant, Bush, and Bronk, no one has come even close to playing Welch's role. Perhaps nobody ever will again.

A Note on the Sources

THE TWO MOST IMPORTANT primary sources for the life of Welch are the three volumes of his *Papers and Addresses,* edited by Walter C. Burket (Baltimore, 1920); and the enormous collection of manuscripts and other papers — seven giant packing cases — in the William H. Welch Library of the Johns Hopkins Medical School. An admirable calendar and catalogue of these "Welch papers," without which they would defy ready consultation, was prepared under the direction of Simon Flexner for use in the writing of his and James Thomas Flexner's *William Henry Welch and the Heroic Age of American Medicine* (New York, 1941). The Flexners also gathered much information, largely embodied in their book, but some of it simply deposited in the Welch papers, through personal interviews and correspondence with those who had known Welch. Many of these people are now dead.

For Welch's associates at Johns Hopkins, Harvey Cushing's *Life of Sir William Osler* (Oxford, 1925) is one of the great biographies in the English language. See also the vivid evocation of Osler by William Sydney Thayer, *Osler and Other Papers* (Baltimore, 1931). W. G. MacCallum's *Willam Stewart Halsted* (Baltimore, 1930) is brief, but on the human side adequate. A life of Howard Kelly is a desideratum; in the meantime, he figures largely in Judith Robinson's *Tom Cullen of Baltimore* (Toronto, 1949), a remarkable biography, with many autobiographical interpolations, of his most notable disciple. Florence R. Sabin's *Franklin Paine Mall* (Baltimore, 1934) is a very perceptive book by one of Mall's best students. John F. Fulton's *Harvey Cushing* (Springfield, Illinois, 1946) contains many vivid glimpses of Welch. Of persons not on the staff at Johns Hopkins, three valuable biographies are: Charles-Edward A. Winslow's *The Life of Hermann M. Biggs* (Philadelphia, 1929), the most important single source for the history of the public health movement in America; Abraham Flexner's *I Remember, The Autobiography of Abraham Flexner* (New York, 1940); and the second edition of Allan Nevins's life of John D. Rockefeller, now called *Study in Power* (New York, 1953).

The official "chronicle" of *The Johns Hopkins Hospital and The Johns Hopkins University School of Medicine*, by Alan M. Chesney, is now in progress; the first volume (Baltimore, 1943) covers the period 1867–1893. An informal history coming down to the immediate past is Bertram M. Bernheim's *The Story of the Johns Hopkins* (New York, 1948) — a very shrewd and pungent book by a member of the staff. The classical panorama of American medical instruction at the beginning of the twentieth century will always remain Abraham Flexner's *Medical Education in the United States and Canada* (New York, 1910).

There is no adequate history of pathology in English. On Virchow, see Irmingard Hasche-Klünder's "Rudolf Virchow, Infektion und Infektionskrankheit, Bakteriologie und Pathologie," *Centaurus*, II (1952), pp. 205-250. On Carl Ludwig's influence in America, see George Rosen's "Carl Ludwig and His American Students," *Bulletin of the History of Medicine*, IV (1936), pp. 609-650. The best account of Cohnheim's laboratory in Welch's time is Carl Julius Salomonsen's "Reminiscences of the Summer Semester, 1877, at Breslau," C. Lilian Temkin, trans. and ed., *Bulletin of the History of Medicine*, XXIV (1950), pp. 333-351.

Two important books by Richard H. Shryock almost exhaust the recent serious literature bearing on American medical history in its long sweep: *The Development of Modern Medicine*, 2d ed. (New York, 1947); and *American Medical Research* (New York, 1947).

Acknowledgments

I SHOULD BE SORRY if the present book were to keep anyone from reading Simon Flexner and James Thomas Flexner's *William Henry Welch and the Heroic Age of American Medicine* (New York: Viking Press, 1941) — one of the notable American biographies. It gives a really spacious portrayal of the detail of Welch's life in a way not possible here, and will bring the reader in touch with another great American, the late Simon Flexner himself. I am greatly indebted throughout to the Flexners; but I have tried to rethink Welch's career from the primary sources, of which the Flexners' book is for certain purposes one.

For the privilege of consulting the Welch papers, I am indebted to Dr. Sanford V. Larkey, librarian of the William H. Welch Library at the Johns Hopkins University. Richard H. Shryock, William H. Welch Professor of the History of Medicine at Johns Hopkins and director of the Institute of the History of Medicine, put every facility at my disposal. I am glad to have worked in this great library and institute, with their many reminders of Welch. I have also a continuing debt to the libraries of Brown University.

The manuscript of this book was read by Professor Oscar Handlin, of Harvard University, editor of the series to which it belongs, and my colleague Professor Edmund S. Morgan, of Brown University. I am grateful for their criticisms, which I have tried, I am afraid very imperfectly, to meet.

DONALD FLEMING

Providence, Rhode Island
1954

Index

William Henry Welch is abbreviated WHW.
See headings Hospitals *and* Universities *for those other than Johns Hopkins.*

ABBOTT, ALEXANDER C., 122, 133
Abel, John J., 100, 105-106
Academy of Surgery (Paris), 5
"Adaptation in Pathological Processes" (WHW), 128-129
Alabama Student, An (Osler), 195
Allbutt, Sir Clifford, 197
American Association for the Advancement of Science, 131
American Medical Association, 132; WHW's presidency, 160
American Red Cross, 192
Antivivisection, origins, 145-147; campaign for Congressional action, 148-149; WHW's reaction to, 148-151
Army Medical Corps (U.S.A.), 82
Association of American Physicians, 131, 149
A.S.P.C.A., 146

Bacillus welchii. *See* Welch bacillus
Bacteriology, origins, 44-45; influence of Cohnheim, Koch, 45, 47-48; early impact in America, 71-73; WHW's study of, 73-76; WHW's researches, 122-124

Baer, Karl Ernst von, 33
Baltimore, significance of WHW's removal to, 70; in 1880's, 77-78; initial response to Johns Hopkins University in, 78-81; WHW and water supply in, 116
Baltimore and Ohio RR., 96, 97, 98
Barker, Lewellys F., early career, 165; advocates full-time, 165; as Osler's successor, 171-172; innovations of, at Hopkins, 172-173; declines to go on full-time, 178
Bassett, John, 21-22
Beers, Clifford, 144-145; and psychiatry at Hopkins, 172-173
"Benefits of the Endowment of Medical Research, The" (WHW), 155
Bergh, Henry, 146-147
Bernard, Claude, 36, 42-43, 194
Biggs, Hermann M., WHW's student, 72; on public health in democracy, 143-144; and Rockefeller Institute, 154, 155; attitude on public health instruction, 181; at international Red Cross Conference, 192

INDEX

Billings, John Shaw, 92; plans for Johns Hopkins medical school, 55; recommends WHW for Hopkins, 65-66; designs hospital plan, 84-86; urges instruction in history of medicine, 115, 194; veterinary research, 122

Blachstein, Arthur G., 127

Bowditch, Henry P., 5

British science, in 19th century, 35; influence on Johns Hopkins, 83-84

Brown-Séquard, C. E., 26

Buckle, Henry T., 18-19

Bull, C. G., 191-192

Buttrick, Wallace, 135; and hookworm campaign, 180; and medicine in China, 186

CANNON, WALTER B., 150-151

Carnegie, Andrew, 68

Carnegie Foundation for the Advancement of Teaching, 173-175

Carnegie Institution of Washington, 131, 157-158

Carrel, Alexis, 133, 189

Carroll, James, 126

Cell theory, in pathology, 42

Chapin, Charles V., 140-141

Charcot, Jean (1825-1893), 26

Charity Organization movement, 138-139

China, medicine in, 186-187

China Medical Board (Rockefeller Foundation), 186

Cobbe, Frances Power, 147

Cohn, Ferdinand, 45, 47; and WHW, 53-54

Cohnheim, Julius, 34, 52, 74; laboratory, 40-41; and Virchow, 43-44; and Koch, 45; Ludwig sends WHW to, 46-47; and bacteriology, 47-48; WHW's research under, 49-51; recommends WHW for Hopkins, 66; on thrombosis, 120-121; on hemorrhagic infarction, 121

Cole, Rufus, 133

Colleges. See Universities

Councilman, W. T., WHW's first assistant, 82, 109, 116, 133; and the malarial crescent, 94, 127

Country Life Commission (1906), 134-135, 180

Cullen, Thomas S., 93-94, 114, 133; research under WHW, 127; on cancer, 145

Cushing, Harvey, 190, 201; on WHW, 3; and Halsted, 113

DARWINISM, WHW's attitude on, 54

Delafield, Francis, 56; and WHW, 28, 58-59, 61-62; haematoxylin stain, 40

Dennis, Frederic, 56, 62; schoolmate of WHW, 30; commends WHW to Gilman, 30; procures appointments for WHW, 58; opposes WHW's removal to Baltimore, 67-70; breaks with WHW, 73

Dewey, John, 103

Diphtheria, 122, 125

Döllinger, Ignaz, 33

Drake, Daniel, 9-10

Draper, John W., 25

EDEMA, PULMONARY, WHW's researches on, 49-51

Ehrlich, Paul, 45; theory of immunity, 135

Eliot, Charles W., 5, 78, 182

Emphysema, 123

Evolution. See Darwinism

"Evolution of Modern Scientific Laboratories, The" (WHW), 195

Expatriatism, and science, 57-58

FATTY DEGENERATION OF HEART, 121-122

Filth theory of disease, 140-142

Fitz, Reginald, 115

Fleming, George, 146

Flexner, Abraham, and John Dewey,

103; report on medical education in U.S., 173-174; report on medical education in Europe, 174-175; and full-time, 175-179; and history of medicine at Johns Hopkins, 196

Flexner, Simon, 126, 133; WHW's assistant, 109; research on diphtheria, 125; director of Rockefeller Institute, 155; and hookworm campaign, 180; and medicine in China, 186

Flint, Austin, Sr., 25; and WHW, 58, 62; supports bacteriology, 71-72

Flügge, Karl, 74, 193

Foot and mouth disease, 126

Franklin, Benjamin, 131, 158

French science, in nineteenth century, 26, 35-37

Freud, Sigmund, 26

Frobenius, Wilhelm, 73

Frosch, Paul, 126

Full-time, genesis of idea, 165; first proposals, 165; WHW's early attitude toward, 166; temperamentally congenial to WHW, 166-168; Osler's opposition to, 169; Abraham Flexner supports, 175-176; open support by WHW, 176-177; issue put to medical faculty, 177-178; WHW's delay in pressing issue, 178-179; plan adopted, 179; effect of controversy on Hopkins, 179-180

GALLINGER, JACOB H., 148-150

Garrett, John Work (1820-1884), 97

Garrett, Mary Elizabeth, 97-99

Garrison, Fielding H., 197

Gates, Frederick T., 155; and genesis of Rockefeller Institute, 152-154; and full-time, 175, 176; and medicine in China, 186

General Education Board, 180; and full-time, 176, 179; and public health instruction, 181; and School of Hygiene at Hopkins, 182; and Wilmer Clinic, 194; endows study of history of medicine at Hopkins, 197-199

Gerhard, W. W., 9-10

Gerhardt, Charles, 35-36

German science, *passim*, 32-56, 71-76; compared with British and French in 19th century, 35-37

Gilchrist, T. C., 127, 133

Gilman, Daniel Coit, 29, 30, 56, 73, 92, 138, 157; and WHW's appointment at Johns Hopkins, 65-67; and benefactresses of Hopkins medical school, 97-99; and Abraham Flexner, 173, 174

Glomerulitis, intracapillary, 120

Gloves, rubber, in surgery, 113-114

Godfrey, Hollis, 189

Goodpasture, Ernest, 133

Gorgas, William C., 134, 190, 192

Gwinn, Mary, 97

HALE, GEORGE ELLERY, 188-189

Halsted, Caroline Hampton (Mrs. W. S.), 113-114, 117

Halsted, William S., 100, 117, 175-176; early career, 63-65; leader of innovations in New York, 64; and local anesthesia, 86-87; becomes cocaine addict, 87-88; goes to Baltimore, 87-88; mature personality, 88; meets Mall, 93; "Halsted suture," 93; versatility of, 105; and Hugh Young, 106; as surgeon, 112-114; as host, 117; and antiseptic surgery, 123-124; relationship with Mall, 162-163; Osler's opinion of, 163, 178; death, 194

Hampton, Caroline. *See* Halsted, Caroline Hampton

Hampton, Wade, 113

Hanselmann's Bar, 116-117

INDEX

Herter, Christian A. (1865-1910), 133; and Rockefeller Institute, 153, 155, 156
Heubner, Johann, 34
His, Wilhelm, Sr., 38
His, Wilhelm, Jr., 193
History of Civilization (Buckle), 18-19
History of medicine, study of, by historical club at Hopkins, 114-115; at Hopkins, 194-199, 201
Holt, L. Emmett (1855-1924), 153, 155
Hookworm disease, 135, 180
Hoover, Herbert, 200, 201
Hopkins, Johns (1795-1873), 29, 81
Hoppe-Seyler, E. F., 33
Hospital, place in university structure, 81-82; architecture, 84-86; administration, 92; role in medical instruction, 106-107
Hospitals. *See also* Johns Hopkins Hospital; Bellevue Hospital (N.Y.), 27-28; Butler Hospital (Providence), 87; Massachusetts General Hospital (Boston), 113; Pennsylvania Hospital (Phila.), 4; Roosevelt Hospital (N.Y.), 64, 87; University Hospital, University of Pennsylvania (Phila.), 5
Howell, William H., early career, 100; goes to Hopkins, 100; at School of Hygiene, 182, 183
Howland, John, 196
Humanism, medical, 197
Hunter, John, 38, 194
Huntington Library, 200
Hurd, Henry M., 91, 98, 111, 138, 159; founds *Hospital Bulletin*, 92
Huxley, T. H., 79, 104; at Johns Hopkins inaugural, 54; and teaching of biology, 83-84; recommends Newell Martin, 84; influence on Mall, 108

IMMUNITY, WHW on, 129; Ehrlich on, 135

Infarction, hemorrhagic, 121
Inflammation, 44, 51-52
"Influence of Louis on American Medicine, The" (Osler), 195
Influential, concept of the, 131-132
Influenza pandemic, 1918-1919, 191
Institute of the History of Medicine, Johns Hopkins, 194-199, 201
International Health Board (Rockefeller Foundation), 193
International Health Commission (Rockefeller Foundation), 180

JACKSON, JAMES, SR., 8
Jackson, James, Jr., 8
Jacobi, Abraham, 28-29, 97, 135
James, Henry, 78, 118
Johns Hopkins Hospital, *passim* 77-118; place in university scheme, 81-82; hospital building, 84-86; administrative structure, 92; role in medical instruction, 106-107; Osler in the wards of, 111-112; surgical traditions, 112-114
Johns Hopkins Hospital Bulletin, The, 92, 114
Johns Hopkins Hospital Historical Club, 114-115, 194-195
Johns Hopkins Medical School, 133, 137, 156; plans for, 55-56; WHW considered for, 65-67; offer to WHW, 67-69; WHW's acceptance, 68-70; local response in Baltimore, 78-81; hospital connection, 81-82; British influence on, 83-84; choice of clinical professors, 86-91; early history, *passim* 96-118; financing of, 96-99; choice of preclinical professors, 100-102; philosophy of instruction, 103-105; versatility of staff, 105-106; nature of instruction, 106-110; distinctive

INDEX

contribution, 110; atmosphere, 110-118; WHW's laboratory, *passim* 119-130; and full-time controversy, 165-180; model for other schools, 174; Institute of History of Medicine at, 194-199, 201

Johns Hopkins Medical Society, 114-115

Johns Hopkins University, 165; and graduate training, 9; opening ceremonies, 54; plans for medical school, 55-56; and Baltimore, 78-81; intellectual role of hospital, 81-82; medical school at, established, 96-102; School of Hygiene established, 182; Institute of History of Medicine, 194-199, 201. *See also* Johns Hopkins Hospital, Johns Hopkins Medical School

Journal of Experimental Medicine, 159

KELLY, HOWARD A., 93, 98, 112, 145, 166, 194; early career, 89-90; goes to Baltimore, 90; Osler's protégé, 90; personality, 90-91; sends gynecology residents to WHW, 94; crisis in his department (1895), 114; and history of medicine, 115; habits of, 116; and Abraham Flexner's report on full-time, 177; acquiesces in full-time, 179

King, Elizabeth, 97

Klebs, Arnold, 198

Klebs-Loeffler bacillus (diphtheria), 122

Koch, Robert, 11, 36, 71, 75; place in history, 44-45; WHW meets, 45, 47; discovery of tubercle bacillus, 72; WHW's teacher, 73-76

Koller, Carl, 87

Kühne, Willy, 66

LABORATORY TRADITION, in Germany, *passim* 32-56; origins, in pathology, in New York, 59-62; in bacteriology, *passim* 71-76; at Johns Hopkins, *passim* 119-130

Laënnec, René, 49

LaFleur, H. A., 127

League of Nations, 192, 193, 201

League of Red Cross Societies, 193

Leffingwell, Albert, 147

Leidy, Joseph, 90

Leuckart, Rudolf, 34; influence on WHW, 54

Lister, Joseph, Lord, 11, 86, 146

Loeffler, Friedrich, 125, 126

Loomis, Alfred L., 72

Louis, Pierre, 28, 38, 129; and the Jacksons, 8; and W. W. Gerhard, 10; historical significance, 10; William Wickham Welch uninfluenced by, 21-22

Ludwig, Carl, 34, 74, 100; physiological institute, 38-40; place in history, 42-43; legacy to students, 45-46; sends WHW to Cohnheim, 46-47; WHW's research, 48-49; for full-time, 165

Lymphosarcoma, 48

MACCALLUM, W. G., 127, 133, 182, 196

McCollum, E. V., 183

Macewen, Sir William, 86

Magendie, François, 42

Mall, Franklin P., 133, 166, 167, 172, 179; meets Halsted, 93; appointment at Johns Hopkins, 100-102; early career, 101-102; philosophy of medical education, 104; methods of teaching, 107-110; and WHW on hemorrhagic infarction, 121; personality, 161; relationship with Halsted, 162; student response to, 162; Osler's attitude toward, 163; relationship with WHW,

Mall *(continued)*
164-165; and genesis of full-time, 165; Osler's farewell to, 171; and Abraham Flexner, 174-175; and full-time at Hopkins, 175-176; death, 194

Manson, Sir Patrick, 136

Martin, H. Newell, 67, 79, 104; role at Hopkins, 82-84; links with WHW, 82-83; end of career, 100; influence continues, 100

Maryland Board of Health, 142, 181

Maryland Club, 78, 117, 159, 175

Maxwell, James Clerk, 84

Medical and Chirurgical Faculty of Maryland, 80

Medical Education in the United States and Canada (Abraham Flexner), 174

Medical research, in Germany, *passim* 32-56, 71-76; at Hopkins, *passim* 119-130; helped by Rockefeller Institute, *passim* 152-160

Medical schools. *See* Universities

Meltzer, Samuel J., 65

Mental health movement, 144-145; and Johns Hopkins, 172-173

Metchnikoff, Elie, 135

Meyer, Adolf, 173

Middlemarch, 129, 202

Morgan, John, 4-6, 8

Müller, Johannes, 36, 43

Murphy, Starr J., 153, 155

NATIONAL ACADEMY OF SCIENCES (U.S.), 132; and World War I, 188

National Research Council, 188-189

National Tuberculosis Association, 144

Naunyn, Bernard, 121-122

Naval Medical School (U.S.), 136

Nightingale, Florence, 85

Noguchi, Hideyo, 126

Numerical method of Louis, 10, 21

Nuttall, G. H. F., 123, 133

OPIE, EUGENE L., 125, 127, 133

Opsonins, 125

Osborn, Henry Fairfield, 60-61

Osler, Grace, Lady (formerly Mrs. S. W. Gross), 97, 188

Osler, Revere, 188, 194

Osler, Sir William, 98, 100, 108, 122, 166, 188; meets WHW, 60-61; appearance, personality, 88-89; goes to Baltimore, 89; reforms hospital administration, 92; least influenced by WHW, 94; versatility, 105; teaching in wards, 106-107; walking the wards, 111-112; and historical club, 115; and medical social service, 116; as host, 117; and antituberculosis campaign, 144; and genesis of Rockefeller Institute, 153; opinion of Mall and Halsted, 163; contrasted with WHW, 168-171; goes to England, 169-171; opposition to full-time, 169, 177-179; favors full-time at McGill, 179; death, 194; as medical historian, 194-195; as medical humanist, 196-197

PANAMA CANAL, 134

Pasteur, Louis, 11, 36, 74

Pathology, history of, in nineteenth century, 42-45; early reception of bacteriology, 47-48; WHW's student researches in, 48-52; impact of bacteriology in America, 71-73; WHW as laboratory director, 119-125; contributions to, of Welch school, 127-128

Pepper, William, Jr., 5

Pettenkofer, Max von, 73-74, 181

Phagocytism, 135

Philanthropy (medical and scientific), significance of, 7-8; Johns Hopkins, 29; Andrew Carnegie, 68, 157; Rockefeller Institute,

INDEX

passim 152-160; Henry Phipps, 172-173; General Education Board, 176-179 (and full-time), 181-182 (and public health instruction), 194 (and Wilmer Clinic), 197-199 (and history of medicine); Rockefeller Foundation and public health instruction, 181-183

Phipps, Henry, 172-173
Pirquet, Clemens von, 176
Pneumococcus, 122
Pneumopathology, 123
Principles and Practice of Medicine (Austin Flint, Sr.), 62
Principles and Practice of Medicine (William Osler), 153
Prudden, T. Mitchell, 133; and WHW, 55-56, 62; as Koch's student, 74-76; on diphtheria, 122; and Rockefeller Institute, 154, 155
Public health instruction, need for, in universities, 181; School of Hygiene at Hopkins, 182-184
Public Health and Marine Hospital Service (U.S.), 134, 143
Public health movement, 140-145, 180

QUIZ, 63-65; run by WHW, 63

"RECENT STUDIES OF IMMUNITY, ON" (WHW), 129
Recklinghausen, F. D. von, 33, 34; WHW's research under, 51-52; on thrombosis, 120-121; on fatty degeneration of heart, 121-122; on adenomyoma of uterus, 127
Reed, Walter, 82, 115, 148; guidance from WHW on yellow fever, 126; research under WHW, 127
Remsen, Ira, 67, 177
Research. *See* Medical research
Rockefeller, John D., Sr., 135; and origins of Rockefeller Institute, 152-153, 155

Rockefeller, John D., Jr., and origins of Rockefeller Institute, 153, 155, 157; and hookworm campaign, 180
Rockefeller Foundation, 180, 181, 182, 183, 186, 193
Rockefeller Institute, 131, 133, 152-154, 155, 156, 159; WHW's contributions to, 156-157; expectations of Rockefellers, 157
Roosevelt, Franklin D., 201
Roosevelt, Theodore, 134, 188
Rose, Wickliffe, and hookworm campaign, 180; and public health instruction, 181

SACCO AND VANZETTI, 201
Salomonsen, Carl, 40, 41, 45, 47
Sarton, George, 198
Schenck, F. von, 34
Schutz, WHW's *Diener*, 109
Seguin, Edward C. (1843-1898), 25, 34, 60; teaches WHW, 26
Shriver, Alfred J., 158, 159
Sigerist, Henry, 199, 201
Singer, Charles, 201
Skull and Bones (Yale society), 20
Smith, Theobald, 155
Social Darwinism, 139-140
Social service, medical, 116
Socialism of hygiene, 142-144, 193
"Some of the Conditions Which Have Influenced the Development of American Medicine" (WHW), 195
Staphylococcus epidermidis albus, 123
Stein, Gertrude, 107, 116, 162
Sternberg, G. M., 82
Stiles, Charles W., 135, 180
Sudhoff, Karl, 199
Surgery at Johns Hopkins, 112-114

THERAPEUTIC NIHILISM, 10, 21-22, 153
Thomas, M. Carey, 96-99

Thrombosis, 120-121
Tuberculosis, campaign against, 144

UNIVERSITIES, COLLEGES, AND MEDICAL SCHOOLS (*see also* Johns Hopkins University and medical school), Bellevue Hospital Medical School, 25, 27, 58, 65; Berlin University, 74; Breslau University, 34, 45, 47, 49, 53-54; Cohnheim's laboratory, 40-41; Bryn Mawr College, 96; California, University of, 133; Cambridge University, 133; Chicago, University of, 101, 165, 176; Clark University, 101; Collège de France, 35; Columbia University, 154 (*see also* Physicians and Surgeons, College of, N. Y.); Cornell University, 29; Göttingen University, 74; Harvard Medical School, 4-6, 96, 100, 133, 156, 164; Leipzig University, 33-34, 48, 74, 199; Ludwig's institute, 38-40; McGill University, 156; Maryland, University of, Medical School, 79, 82; Michigan, University of, Medical School, 100, 101, 105; Munich University, 73-74, 181; New York University Medical School, 25, 27; Northwestern University Medical School, 5; Oxford University, 169; Peking Union Medical College, 136; modernization, 186-187; Pennsylvania, University of, Medical School, 5, 89-90, 96, 105, 133, 155 (*see also* Philadelphia, College of); Philadelphia, College of, Medical School, 4-5; Physicians and Surgeons, College of (Baltimore), 79; Physicians and Surgeons, College of (N. Y.), 133; WHW as student, 24-27; repute, 25; no opening for WHW at, 58-59; new laboratory at, 61-62; Rochester, University of, 133; Sheffield Scientific School (Yale University), 22-23; WHW as student, 24; Sorbonne, 35; Strassburg University, 33, 34, 51-52; Tulane University Medical School, 136; Vienna University, 34; Washington University (St. Louis), 133; Yale College, 24, 30, 63; WHW as student, 18-20; Yale Medical School, 12, 24, 133; Yale University (*see* Sheffield Scientific School, Yale College, Yale Medical School); Zurich University, 96
University Club (Baltimore), 117, 159

VENABLE, RICHARD M., 158, 159
Virchow, Rudolf, 28, 36, 71; applies cell theory to pathology, 42; and von Recklinghausen, Cohnheim, and Weigert, 43-44; on inflammation, 44, 51-52; Ludwig diverts WHW from, 46-47; concept of thrombosis, 120-121
Voegtlin, Carl, 127

WAGNER, ERNEST, 34, 53, 55, 100; guides WHW's research, 48
Walcott, Emma Welch (Mrs. Stuart Walcott, WHW's sister), 13, 54, 159; friendship with WHW, 15-18; marriage, 27; favors European study, 30; death, 158
Walcott, Stuart (WHW's brother-in-law), 27, 30, 68, 158
Waldeyer, Wilhelm, 33, 53
Weber, Ernst von, 147
Weigert, Carl, 34, 40, 47, 53; and Virchow, 44; and Koch, 45; and academic anti-Semitism, 74
Welch, Benjamin (WHW's grandfather), 12
Welch, Elizabeth Loveland (WHW's grandmother), 12-16, 18

INDEX

Welch, Emeline Collin (WHW's mother), 13

Welch, Emily Sedgwick (WHW's stepmother), 18, 69; favors European study, 31; and move to Baltimore, 68; death, 158

Welch, Emma. *See* Walcott, Emma Welch

Welch, Hopestill (WHW's great-grandfather), 12

Welch, William Henry

EARLY LIFE AND SCHOOLING, necessary conditions for his career, 6-11; ancestors, 12; parents and grandmother, 12-14; home life as child, 14-16; early schooling, 15-17; conversion experience, 16-18; at Yale College, 18-21; choice of career, 21-22; at Sheffield School (Yale), 22-24; at College of Physicians and Surgeons (N. Y.), 24-27; and Edward C. Seguin, 26; prosector, 26-27; intern at Bellevue, 27-29; and Francis Delafield, 28; first aspirations toward Hopkins, 29-30

EUROPEAN STUDY AND RESEARCH, to Europe for study, 30-31; teachers and studies, 33-34, 37-41; and Ludwig, 45-47; and Cohnheim, 47-48; first researches, 48-52; opinion of Germany, 52-54; and Darwinism, 54; prospects at Johns Hopkins, 55-56; return to America, 57; laboratory at Bellevue, 59-61; other New York activities, 62-63; failure to do research, 65; appointed to Hopkins, 65-69, 70; awareness of bacteriology, 71-73; return to Germany, 73; first courses in bacteriology, 73-74; with Koch, 74-76

START OF CAREER AT JOHNS HOPKINS, move to Baltimore, 78; and local sensitivities, 80-81; affinities with faculty of philosophy, 81-82; and Newell Martin, 82-83; secures appointment of Halsted, 86-88; influence on clinical colleagues, 93-95; opposition to medical coeducation, 98; role in choice of preclinical professors, 100-102; philosophy of medical instruction, 104-105; as classroom instructor, 108-110; significance of work, 110; and Hopkins atmosphere, 116-118; personal researches in Baltimore, 119-125; Welch bacillus, 122-123; place in creative tradition, 124; relationship with students, 124-127, 128; withdrawal from research, 128-130

DEVELOPMENT AS AN INFLUENTIAL, positions of power held, 131-132; placing of his students, 133; role in public life, 134-135; routine tasks as Influential, 135-137; novelty of his position, 137-138; on organized charity, 138-139; and Social Darwinism, 139-140; on filth theory of disease, 140-141; socialism of hygiene, 142-143; on public health and democracy, 143-145; and antivivisection, 145-150; opposed to lay group supporting vivisection, 150-151; and Rockefeller Institute, 154-157; and Carnegie Institution of Washington, 157-158; private life in maturity, 158-160

RELATIONSHIP WITH OSLER, relationship with Mall, 164-165; attitude toward full-time, 166-168; departure of Osler, 171; choice of Osler's successor, 171-172; secures endowment of psychiatric instruction, 172-173; open support for full-time, 176-

INDEX

Welch *(continued)*
177; delay in initiating full-time, 178-179; and School of Hygiene, 180-183

WORLD WAR I AND AFTER, outbreak of World War I, 185-186; studies medical instruction in China, 186-187; founding of National Research Council, 188; to Europe in 1916, 188-189; crisis for National Research Council, 189; war services, 190-191; Welch bacillus in war, 191-192; international Red Cross proposals, 192-193; Germany in the 1920's, 193; death of colleagues, 194; takes up history of medicine, 194-199; 80th birthday, 199-200; choice of successor in history of medicine, 201; last illness and death, 201-202

Welch, William Wickham (WHW's father), 12-14, 54, 121; second marriage, 18; professional standing, 21-22; and WHW's European study, 30-31; and WHW's move to Baltimore, 68; death, 158

Welch bacillus, discovery of, 123; in World War I, 191-192

Whipple, George H., 125-126, 133

Williams, J. Whitridge, 94, 133

Wilmer, William H., 194

Wilson, Woodrow, 188, 192; WHW's attitude toward, 185

Winternitz, Milton C., 133

Women's Fund Committee, for Johns Hopkins Medical School, 97-98

World War I, 185-193

Wright, Sir Almroth, 125, 189

YOUNG, HUGH, 106; recollection of WHW, 158-159

ZINSSER, HANS, 133